POCKET GUIDE TO
Clinical Microbiology

2ND EDITION

2ND EDITION

POCKET GUIDE TO

Clinical
Microbiology

Patrick R. Murray, PH.D., ABMM

Professor, Pathology and Medicine
Director, Clinical Microbiology Laboratories
Washington University Medical Center
St. Louis, Missouri

ASM
PRESS

WASHINGTON, D.C.

Copyright   1998 American Society for Microbiology
             1325 Massachusetts Avenue, N.W.
             Washington, DC 20005

Library of Congress Cataloging-in-Publication Data

Murray, Patrick R.
  Pocket guide to clinical microbiology/Patrick R. Murray. —
2nd ed.
     p.   cm.
  Rev. ed. of: ASM pocket guide to clinical
microbiology/Patrick R. Murray. c1996.
  Includes bibliographical references and index.
  ISBN 1-55581-137-X (softcover)
  1. Medical microbiology—Handbooks, manuals, etc.
I. Murray, Patrick R. ASM pocket guide to clinical
microbiology.   II. Title.
  [DNLM: 1. Microbiology handbooks.
2. Microbiological Techniques handbooks.   3. Antibiosis
handbooks.   4. Microbial Sensitivity Tests handbooks.
QW 39 M983p 1998]
QR46.M92   1998
616 .01—dc21
DNLM/DLC
for Library of Congress   96-21385
                                                      CIP

10 9 8 7 6 5 4 3 2 1

To Melissa
for her inspiration, support, and
patience during the preparation
of this book

Contents

SECTION 6
Vaccines, Antibiotics, and Susceptibility Testing 243

Preface

The first edition of the *Pocket Guide to Clinical Microbiology* was designed to be a convenient reference source for commonly asked questions in clinical microbiology. Toward this goal the *Pocket Guide* successfully addressed questions about basic microbiology; specimen collection, transport, and processing; identification of clinically important microbes; antibiotics, susceptibility patterns, and susceptibility test methods; interpretation of test results; and trends in infectious diseases. With the experience of using this resource guide for the past 2 years, I have found what worked well and what fell short. In this edition I have attempted to update, correct, reorganize, and supplement the original presentation. Although the basic eight sections have been retained, the information within each section has been extensively changed. In some cases the information has been reorganized, such as moving the morphological classification of filamentous fungi from the taxonomy section to the identification section and then expanding this material to practical guidelines for the identification of these fungi. In other sections the presentation has been extensively expanded, such as the coverage of organisms responsible for infectious diseases (section 2), recommendations for the collection (section 3) or processing (section 4) of specimens for specific microbes, summary of antimicrobial susceptibility patterns for common pathogens (section 6), and interpretation of immunodiagnostic tests (section 7). Finally, new information has been added throughout the *Pocket Guide*, particularly for identification of common organisms (section 5), immunization recommendations for U.S. inhabitants and travelers (section 6), and an index. It is my hope that each change will represent an improvement, providing factual information in an easy-to-use format.

No individual can successfully complete a project of this magnitude without the help of many others. In the first edition I thanked the microbiologists who were responsible for my early training and my colleagues who make my job so easy now. My praise of those individuals will always be there. I also thank my secretary, Linda Dickey, who seems to balance a number of tasks without ever making a mistake. Finally, I thank the ASM staff for their help with this project, particularly Susan Birch, Production Manager for ASM Press, who once again reaffirmed my confidence in her skills as an editor, therapist, and politician.

Taxonomic Classification of Medically Important Microorganisms

Phenotypic classification of organisms (e.g., microscopic and macroscopic morphologies, biochemical properties, antigenic composition) has largely been replaced by genotypic analysis (e.g., DNA homology, rRNA sequencing). Not only can this approach precisely define relationships among organisms, revealing previously unrecognized similarities and differences, but also unculturable organisms can be detected and identified. Since the first edition of this text, a number of organisms have been discovered, renamed, or reclassified. The following section represents what I believe is an accurate review of the current status of microbial taxonomy. It must be recognized that some of the relationships presented in the following tables are provisional and may be changed in the future. Likewise, names are certain to be modified and new organisms will be identified. This underscores the fact that taxonomic classification is an actively evolving science that should form the foundation of our expanding knowledge of clinical microbiology.

The information in this section was collected from numerous published articles (particularly in the *International Journal of Systematic Bacteriology*), as well as from the reference texts cited in the Bibliography.

Taxonomic Classification of Bacteria

Eubacteria have been subdivided into at least 11 divisions, including 5 with medically important organisms.

1. Division: Proteobacteria
  Subdivision: Alpha subclass
    Subgroup 1
      Genus. *Brevundimonas*
    Subgroup 2
      Family. *Bartonellaceae*
        Genus. *Bartonella*
      Family. *Rickettsiaceae*
        Genus. *Rickettsia*
          Typhus group
          Spotted fever group
        Genus. *Orientia*
        Genus. *Ehrlichia*
          E. canis group

E. phagocytophila group
E. sennetsu group
Genus. *Cowdria*
Genus. *Anaplasma*
Genus. *Neorickettsia*
Uncertain classification
Genus. *Brucella*
Genus. *Agrobacterium*
Genus. *Ochrobactrum*
Subdivision: Beta subclass
Subgroup 1
Genus. *Burkholderia*
Subgroup 2
Family. *Neisseriaceae*
Genus. *Eikenella*
Genus. *Kingella*
Genus. *Neisseria*
Genus. *Simonsiella*
Family. *Alcaligenaceae*
Genus. *Alcaligenes*
Genus. *Bordetella*
Uncertain classification
Genus. *Chromobacterium*
Subgroup 3
Family. *Comamonadaceae*
Genus. *Acidovorax*
Genus. *Comamonas*
Genus. *Hydrogenophaga*
Subdivision: Delta subclass
Genus. *Bdellovibrio*
Genus. *Desulfobacter*
Genus. *Desulfovibrio*
Genus. *Myxococcus*
Subdivision: Gamma subclass
Subgroup 1
Family. *Legionellaceae*
Genus. *Legionella*
Uncertain classification
Genus. *Coxiella*
Genus. *Francisella*
Genus. *Wolbachia*
Subgroup 2
Family. *Enterobacteriaceae*

Genus. *Cedecea*
Genus. *Citrobacter*
Genus. *Edwardsiella*
Genus. *Enterobacter*
Genus. *Escherichia*
Genus. *Ewingella*
Genus. *Hafnia*
Genus. *Klebsiella*
Genus. *Kluyvera*
Genus. *Leclercia*
Genus. *Moellerella*
Genus. *Morganella*
Genus. *Pantoea*
Genus. *Proteus*
Genus. *Providencia*
Genus. *Salmonella*
Genus. *Serratia*
Genus. *Shigella*
Genus. *Tatumella*
Genus. *Yersinia*
Family. *Vibrionaceae*
Genus. *Listonella*
Genus. *Photobacterium*
Genus. *Shewanella*
Genus. *Vibrio*
Family. *Pasteurellaceae*
Genus. *Actinobacillus*
Genus. *Haemophilus*
Genus. *Pasteurella*
Family. *Aeromonadaceae*
Genus. *Aeromonas*
Uncertain classification
Genus. *Plesiomonas*
Subgroup 3
Family. *Pseudomonadaceae*
Genus. *Pseudomonas*
Family. *Moraxellaceae*
Genus. *Acinetobacter*
Genus. *Branhamella*
Genus. *Moraxella*
Uncertain classification
Genus. *Stenotrophomonas*

Subgroup 4
> Family. *Cardiobacteriaceae*
>> Genus. *Cardiobacterium*
>> Genus. *Dichelobacter*
>> Genus. *Suttonella*

Subdivision: Epsilon subclass
> Family. *Campylobacteraceae*
>> Genus. *Arcobacter*
>> Genus. *Campylobacter*
> Uncertain classification
>> Genus. *Helicobacter*
>> Genus. *Wolinella*

2. Division: "Gram-positive" bacteria
  Subdivision 1: Gram-negative anaerobes
> Family. *Veillonellaceae*
>> Genus. *Acidaminococcus*
>> Genus. *Megasphaera*
>> Genus. *Veillonella*
> Uncertain classification
>> Genus. *Selenomonas*
>> Genus. *Sporamusa*

  Subdivision 2: *Heliobacterium*
  Subdivision 3: Bacteria with low G+C mol%
> Order. *Bacillales*
> Family. *Bacillaceae*
>> Genus. *Alicyclobacillus*
>> Genus. *Aneurinibacillus*
>> Genus. *Bacillus*
>>> *B. subtilis* group
>>> *B. cereus* group (includes *B. anthracis*)
>>> *B. sphaericus* group
>> Genus. *Brevibacillus*
>> Genus. *Gemella*
>> Genus. *Listeria*
>> Genus. *Paenibacillus*
>> Genus. *Planococcus*
>> Genus. *Staphylococcus*
>> Genus. *Virgibacillus*
> Family. *Streptococcaceae*
>> Genus. *Enterococcus*
>> Genus. *Lactococcus*
>> Genus. *Streptococcus*

Family. *Lactobacillaceae*
  Genus. *Lactobacillus*
  Genus. *Leuconostoc*
  Genus. *Pediococcus*
Family. *Peptococcaceae*
  Genus: *Atopobium*
  Genus: *Coprococcus*
  Genus: *Peptococcus*
  Genus: *Peptostreptococcus*
  Genus: *Ruminococcus*
  Genus: *Sarcina*
Uncertain affiliation
  Genus. *Aerococcus*
  Genus. *Kurthia*
Order. *Clostriadiales*
Family. *Clostridiaceae* I
  Genus. *Clostridium* (e.g., *C. perfringens*,
    C. butyricum)
Family. *Clostridiaceae* II
  Genus. *Clostridium* (e.g., *C. difficile*)
  Genus. *Eubacterium*
  Genus. *Peptostreptococcus* (i.e., *P. anaerobius*)
Family. *Clostridiaceae* III
  Genus. *Clostridium* (e.g., *C. sphenoides*)
Family. *Clostridiaceae* IV
  Genus. *Clostridium* (e.g., *C. innocuum*,
    C. ramosum)
  Genus. *Erysipelothrix*
  Genus. *Lactobacillus* (*L. catenaforme*)
Order. *Mycoplasmatales*
Family. Mycoplasmataceae
  Genus. *Mycoplasma*
  Genus. *Ureaplasma*
Order. *Entomoplasmatales*
Family. *Entomoplasmataceae*
  Genus. *Entomoplasma*
  Genus. *Mesoplasma*
Family. *Spiroplasmataceae*
  Genus. *Spiroplasma*
Order. *Acholeplasmatales*
Family. *Acholeplasmataceae*
  Genus. *Acholeplasma*
Order. *Anaeroplasmatales*

Family. *Anaeroplasmataceae*
    Genus. *Anaeroplasma*
    Genus. *Asteroleplasma*
Subdivision 4: Bacteria with high G+C mol%
Order. *Actinomycetales*
Suborder. *Micromonosporineae*
    Family. *Micromonosporaceae*
        Genus. *Actinoplanes*
        Genus. *Catellatospora*
        Genus. *Dactylosporangium*
        Genus. *Glycomyces*
        Genus. *Micromonospora*
        Genus. *Pilimelia*
Suborder. *Frankineae*
    Family. *Acidothermaceae*
    Family. *Frankiaceae*
    Family. *Geodermatophilaceae*
    Family. *Microsphaeraceae*
    Family. *Sporichthyaceae*
Suborder. *Pseudonocardineae*
    Family. *Pseudonocardiaceae*
        Genus. *Actinopolyspora*
        Genus. *Amycolata*
        Genus. *Amycolatopsis*
        Genus. *Pseudonocardia*
        Genus. *Saccharomonospora*
        Genus. *Saccharopolyspora*
        Genus. *Saccharothrix*
Suborder. *Streptomycineae*
    Family. *Streptomycetaceae*
        Genus. *Streptomyces*
Suborder. *Corynebacterineae*
    Family. *Corynebacteriaceae*
        Genus. *Corynebacterium*
        Genus. *Dietzia*
        Genus. *Turicella*
    Family. *Nocardiaceae*
        Genus. *Gordona*
        Genus. *Nocardia*
        Genus. *Rhodococcus*
        Genus. *Tsukamurella*
    Family. *Mycobacteriaceae*
        Genus. *Mycobacterium*

Family. *Dietziaceae*
Suborder. *Micrococcineae*
Family. *Intrasporangiaceae*
Family. *Dermatophilaceae*
Family. *Micrococcaceae*
Genus. *Arthrobacter*
Genus. *Micrococcus*
Family. *Promicromonosporaceae*
Family. *Cellulomonadaceae*
Genus. *Cellulomonas*
Genus. *Oerskovia*
Family. *Microbacteriaceae*
Genus. *Aureobacterium*
Genus. *Microbacterium*
Suborder. *Actinomycineae*
Family. *Actinomycetaceae*
Genus. *Actinomyces*
Genus. *Arcanobacterium*
Genus. *Mobiluncus*
Genus. *Rothia*
Genus. *Stomatococcus*
Suborder. *Propionibacterineae*
Family. *Propionibacteriaceae*
Family. *Nocardioidaceae*
Suborder. *Streptosporangineae*
Family. *Streptosporangiaceae*
Genus. *Microbispora*
Genus. *Microtetraspora*
Genus. *Streptosporangium*
Family. *Thermomonosporaceae*
Genus. *Actinomadura*
Genus. *Thermomonospora*
Family. *Nocardiopsaceae*
Suborder. *Glycomycineae*
Family. *Glycomycetaceae*
Order. *Bifidobacteriales*
Family. *Bifidobacteriaceae*

3. Division: Spirochaetes
Order. *Spirochaetales*
Family. *Spirochaetaceae*
Genus. *Borrelia*
Genus. *Cristispira*

Genus. *Serpulina*
Genus. *Spirochaeta*
Genus. *Treponema*
Family. *Leptospiraceae*
Genus. *Leptonema*
Genus. *Leptospira*
Genus. *Turneria*

4. Division: Aerobic and anaerobic bacilli in RNA superfamily V

Subgroup 1

Family. *Bacteroidaceae*
Genus. *Bacteroides*
Genus. *Bilophila*
Genus. *Porphyromonas*
Genus. *Prevotella*
Uncertain classification
Genus. *Fusobacterium*
Genus. *Leptotrichia*

Subgroup 2

Uncertain classification
Genus. *Capnocytophaga*
Genus. *Cytophaga*
Genus. *Flexibacter*
Genus. *Saprospira*
Genus. *Sporocytophaga*

5. Division: Chlamydiae

Order. *Chlamydiales*
Family. *Chlamydiaceae*
Genus. *Chlamydia*

Taxonomic Classification of Human Viruses

Single-stranded, nonenveloped RNA viruses

Caliciviridae	*Calicivirus*	Human calicivirus, Norwalk virus, Norwalk-like viruses
Astroviridae	*Astrovirus*	Astrovirus
Picornaviridae	*Aphthovirus*	Foot-and-mouth disease virus

	Cardiovirus	Encephalomyo-carditis virus
	Enterovirus	Coxsackievirus groups A and B, echoviruses, enterovirus, poliovirus
	Hepatovirus	Hepatitis A virus
	Rhinovirus	Rhinovirus
	Unnamed genus	Echovirus

Single-stranded, enveloped RNA viruses

Arenaviridae	*Arenavirus*	Lymphocytic choriomeningitis (LCM) virus, Lassa fever virus, Junin virus, Machupo virus, Guanarito virus, Sabia virus
Bunyaviridae	*Bunyavirus*	Bunyamwera virus, California encephalitis virus, La Crosse virus
	Hantavirus	Hantaan virus
	Nairovirus	Crimean-Congo hemorrhagic fever virus
	Phlebovirus	Rift Valley fever virus
Coronaviridae	*Coronavirus*	Coronavirus
	Totovirus	Berne virus
Filoviridae	*Filovirus*	Ebola virus, Marburg virus
Flaviviridae	*Flavivirus*	Yellow fever virus, dengue

		virus, St. Louis encephalitis virus
	Hepacivirus	Hepatitis C virus
Orthomyxo-viridae	*Influenzavirus*	Influenza virus, types A, B, and C
Paramyxoviridae *Paramyxo-virinae*	*Morbillivirus*	Measles virus
	Paramyxovirus	Paramyxovirus, Sendai virus
	Rubulavirus	Mumps virus
Pneumovirinae	*Pneumovirus*	Respiratory syncytial virus (RSV)
Retroviridae	HTLV-BLV group	Human T-cell lymphotropic virus (HTLV) types I and II
	Lentivirus	Human immuno-deficiency virus (HIV) types 1 and 2
	Spumavirinae	Human (foamy virus) spuma-virus
Rhabdoviridae	*Lyssavirus*	Rabies virus
	Vesiculovirus	Vesicular stomatitis virus
Togaviridae	*Alphavirus*	Sindbis virus, Eastern equine encephalitis (EEE) virus, Western equine encephalitis (WEE) virus, Venezuelan

		encephalitis virus, Semliki Forest virus
	Rubivirus	Rubella virus

Double-stranded, nonenveloped RNA viruses

Reoviridae	*Coltivirus*	Colorado tick fever virus
	Reovirus	Reovirus
	Rotavirus	Rotavirus

Single-stranded, nonenveloped DNA viruses

Parvoviridae	*Dependovirus*	Adeno-associated virus
	Erythrovirus	B19 virus

Double-stranded, nonenveloped DNA viruses

Adenoviridae	*Mastadenovirus*	Adenovirus
Papovaviridae	*Papillomavirus*	Papillomavirus
	Polyomavirus	JC virus, BK virus

Double-stranded, enveloped DNA viruses

Hepadnaviridae	*Orthohepadna-virus*	Hepatitis B virus
Herpesviridae *Alphaherpes-virinae*	*Simplexvirus*	Herpes simplex virus (HSV)
	Varicellovirus	Varicella-zoster virus (VZV)
Betaherpes-virinae	*Cytomegalovirus*	Cytomegalovirus (CMV)
	Roseolovirus	Human herpesvirus 6
Gamma-herpesvirinae	*Lympho-cryptovirus*	Epstein-Barr virus (EBV)

Poxviridae	*Avipoxvirus*	Fowlpox virus
	Molluscipoxvirus	Molluscum contagiosum virus
	Orthopoxvirus	Vaccinia virus, smallpox virus, cowpox virus, monkeypox virus
	Parapoxvirus	Orf virus
	Suipoxvirus	Swinepox virus

Taxonomic Classification of Fungi

Division. Zygomycotina (lower fungi)
    Class. Zygomycetes
        Order. Mucorales
            Genus. *Apophysomyces*
            Genus. *Absidia*
            Genus. *Cokeromyces*
            Genus. *Cunninghamella*
            Genus. *Mucor*
            Genus. *Rhizomucor*
            Genus. *Rhizopus*
            Genus. *Saksenaea*
            Genus. *Syncephalastrum*
        Order. Entomophthorales
            Genus. *Basidiobolus*
            Genus. *Conidiobolus*

Division. Ascomycotina (higher fungi)
    Class. Ascomycetes
        Order. Endomycetales
            Genus. *Saccharomyces*
            Genus. *Pichia* (teleomorph stage of some *Candida* spp.)
        Order. Onygenales
            Genus. *Arthroderma* (teleomorph stage of *Microsporum* and *Trichophyton*)
            Genus. *Ajellomyces* (teleomorph stage of *Blastomyces* and *Histoplasma*)
        Order. Eurotiales

Genus. *Emericella* (teleomorph stage of
some *Aspergillus*)
Genus. *Eurotium* (teleomorph stage of
some *Aspergillus*)
Genus. *Pseudallescheria* (teleomorph stage
of *Scedosporium*)
Order. Sphaeriales
Genus. *Chaetomium*
Genus. *Neurospora* (*Chrysonilia*)
Order. Pneumocystidales
Genus. *Pneumocystis*

Division. Basidiomycotina
Class. Basidiomycetes
Order. Agaricales
Order. Filobasidiales
Genus. *Filobasidiella* (teleomorphs of
Cryptococcus)

Division. Deuteromycotina (Fungi Imperfecti)
Class. Deuteromycetes
Subclass. Blastomycetes
Order. Cryptococcales
Genus. *Candida*
Genus. *Cryptococcus*
Genus. *Hansenula*
Genus. *Malassezia*
Genus. *Rhodotorula*
Genus. *Trichosporon*
Subclass. Hyphomycetes
Order. Moniliales
Family. Moniliaceae
Genus. *Acremonium*
Genus. *Arthrographis*
Genus. *Aspergillus*
Genus. *Beauveria*
Genus. *Blastomyces*
Genus. *Chrysonilia*
Genus. *Chrysosporium*
Genus. *Coccidioides*
Genus. *Emmonsia*
Genus. *Epidermophyton*
Genus. *Fusarium*
Genus. *Geotrichum*

Genus. *Gliocladium*
Genus. *Histoplasma*
Genus. *Lecythophora*
Genus. *Microsporum*
Genus. *Paecilomyces*
Genus. *Penicillium*
Genus. *Paracoccidioides*
Genus. *Scopulariopsis*
Genus. *Scytalidium*
Genus. *Sepedonium*
Genus. *Sporothrix*
Genus. *Sporotrichum*
Genus. *Trichophyton*
Genus. *Trichoderma*
Genus. *Trichothecium*
Genus. *Tritirachium*
Genus. *Verticillium*
Family. Dematiaceae
Genus. *Alternaria*
Genus. *Arthrinium*
Genus. *Aureobasidium*
Genus. *Bipolaris*
Genus. *Botrytis*
Genus. *Cladosporium*
Genus. *Curvularia*
Genus. *Drechlera*
Genus. *Epicoccum*
Genus. *Exserohilum*
Genus. *Exophiala*
Genus. *Fonsecaea*
Genus. *Helminthosporium*
Genus. *Madurella*
Genus. *Nigrospora*
Genus. *Phialophora*
Genus. *Pithomyces*
Genus. *Rhinocladiella*
Genus. *Scedosporium*
Genus. *Scolecobasidium*
Genus. *Ulocladium*
Genus. *Wangiella*
Genus. *Xylohypha*
Subclass. Coelomycetes
Order. Sphaeropsidales

Genus. *Phoma*
Genus. *Nattrassia*

Taxonomic Classification of Parasites

PROTOZOA
Phylum. Sarcomastigophora
  Subphylum. Mastigophora (flagellates)
          Genus. *Chilomastix* (intestinal)
          Genus. *Dientamoeba* (intestinal)
          Genus. *Enteromonas* (intestinal)
          Genus. *Giardia* (intestinal)
          Genus. *Leishmania* (tissues)
          Genus. *Retortamonas* (intestinal)
          Genus. *Trichomonas* (intestinal, urogenital, oral)
          Genus. *Trypanosoma* (blood, tissues)
  Subphylum. Sarcodina (amoebae)
          Genus. *Acanthamoeba* (free-living)
          Genus. *Balamuthia* (free-living)
          Genus. *Blastocystis* (intestinal)
          Genus. *Endolimax* (intestinal)
          Genus. *Entamoeba* (intestinal)
          Genus. *Iodamoeba* (intestinal)
          Genus. *Naegleria* (free-living)

Phylum. Ciliophora (ciliates)
          Genus. *Balantidium* (intestinal)

Phylum. Apicomplexa (apicomplexans)
      Subclass. Coccidia
          Genus. *Cryptosporidium* (intestinal)
          Genus. *Cyclospora* (intestinal)
          Genus. *Isospora* (intestinal)
          Genus. *Plasmodium* (blood)
          Genus. *Sarcocystis* (intestinal, extraintestinal)
          Genus. *Toxoplasma* (extraintestinal)
      Subclass. Piroplasmea
          Genus. *Babesia* (blood)

Phylum. Microspora (microsporidia)
          Genus. *Encephalitozoon* (intestinal, extraintestinal)
          Genus. *Enterocytozoon* (intestinal)

Genus. *Nosema* (extraintestinal)
Genus. *Pleistophora* (extraintestinal)
Genus. *Trachipleistophora* (extraintestinal)
Genus. *Vittaforma* (extraintestinal)
Genus. Unclassified microsporidia
(extraintestinal)

HELMINTHS
Phylum. Nematoda (roundworms)
Class. Adenophorea (Aphasmidia)
Genus. *Capillaria* (visceral larva migrans; tissues)
Genus. *Trichinella* (tissues)
Genus. *Trichuris* (whipworm; intestinal)
Class. Secernentia (Phasmidia)
Genus. *Ancylostoma* (Old World hookworm; intestinal, extraintestinal)
Genus. *Angiostrongylus* (rat lungworm; tissues)
Genus. *Anisakis* (herringworm disease; intestinal, extraintestinal)
Genus. *Ascaris* (roundworm; intestinal, extraintestinal)
Genus. *Brugia* (lymphatic filaria)
Genus. *Dirofilaria* (dog heartworm; pulmonary tissues)
Genus. *Dracunculus* (Guinea worm; cutaneous tissues)
Genus. *Enterobius* (pinworm; intestinal)
Genus. *Eustrongylides* (extraintestinal)
Genus. *Gnathostoma* (visceral larva migrans; tissues)
Genus. *Loa* (African eye worm; blood and tissues)
Genus. *Mansonella* (dermal filaria)
Genus. *Necator* (New World tapeworm; intestinal)
Genus. *Onchocerca* (tissue filaria)
Genus. *Strongyloides* (threadworm; intestinal)
Genus. *Toxocara* (dog or cat roundworm; visceral larva migrans; tissues)
Genus. *Trichostrongylus* (intestinal)
Genus. *Wuchereria* (lymphatic filaria)

Phylum. Platyhelminthes (flatworms)

    Class. Cestoidea (tapeworms)

        Genus. *Diphyllobothrium* (fish tapeworm; intestinal)

        Genus. *Dipylidium* (pumpkin seed tapeworm; intestinal)

        Genus. *Echinococcus* (hydatid disease; extraintestinal)

        Genus. *Hymenolepis* (dwarf tapeworm; intestinal)

        Genus. *Spirometra* (sparganosis; extraintestinal)

        Genus. *Taenia* (beef and pork tapeworms, intestinal; cysticercosis, extraintestinal)

    Class. Trematoda (flukes)

        Genus. *Clonorchis* (liver fluke)

        Genus. *Dicrocoelium* (liver fluke)

        Genus. *Echinostoma* (intestinal fluke)

        Genus. *Fasciola* (liver fluke)

        Genus. *Fasciolopsis* (intestinal fluke)

        Genus. *Gastrodiscoides* (intestinal fluke)

        Genus. *Haplorchis* (intestinal fluke)

        Genus. *Heterophyes* (intestinal fluke)

        Genus. *Metagonimus* (intestinal fluke)

        Genus. *Metorchis* (liver fluke)

        Genus. *Nanaphyetus* (intestinal fluke)

        Genus. *Neodiplostomum* (intestinal fluke)

        Genus. *Opisthorchis* (liver fluke)

        Genus. *Paragonimus* (lung fluke)

        Genus. *Phaneropsolus* (intestinal fluke)

        Genus. *Prosthodendrium* (intestinal fluke)

        Genus. *Pygidiopsis* (intestinal fluke)

        Genus. *Schistosoma* (blood fluke)

        Genus. *Stellantchasmus* (intestinal fluke)

ARTHROPODS

Phylum. Arthropoda

    Class. Diplopoda (millipedes)

    Class. Chilopoda (centipedes)

    Class. Crustacea (crustaceans)

      Order. Copepoda (copepods)

      Order. Decapoda (crabs, crayfish)

    Class. Insecta (insects)

Order. Anoplura (lice)
Order. Hemiptera (bedbugs, kissing bugs)
Order. Siphonaptera (fleas)
Order. Dictyoptera (cockroaches)
Order. Hymenoptera (ants, wasps, bees)
Order. Coleoptera (beetles)
Order. Diptera (flies, mosquitos, midges)
Order. Lepidoptera (moths, butterflies, caterpillars)
Class. Arachnida (arachnids)
Subclass. Scorpiones (scorpions)
Subclass. Araneae (spiders)
Subclass. Acari (ticks, mites, chiggers)
Class. Pentastomida (tongue worms)

Indigenous and Pathogenic Microbes of Humans

Humans are exposed to microbes at birth, which leads to one of three outcomes: transient colonization, persistent colonization, or pathogenic interaction. The majority of organisms are unable to become established on the skin or mucosal surfaces and are considered an insignificant finding when recovered in clinical specimens. Examples include the molds and many of the nonfermentative gram-negative bacilli that can be isolated in soil, vegetation, water, and food products. These organisms are unable to compete with the normal microbial population of the body or cannot survive on the skin surface.

Other organisms are able to establish long-term residency on or in the human body. The successes of these interactions are influenced by complex microbial and host factors (e.g., favorable environment [pH, atmosphere, moisture, available nutrients], ability to adhere to surfaces, resistance to bacteriocins, antibiotics, and phagocytic cells, etc.). These microbes generally exist in a symbiotic relationship with their human host and only produce disease when they invade normally sterile body sites such as tissues and body fluids. Table 2.1 is a listing of the organisms most commonly recovered from the body surfaces of healthy individuals. This table is intended to serve as an interpretive guideline for cultured specimens. It should be remembered that many organisms cannot be detected when present in a mixed population (typical of many body sites). Additionally, as the taxonomic classification of microbes is updated and more sophisticated identification systems are introduced, our understanding of the prevalence of organisms at specific body sites can change. The quantitative and qualitative presence of specific microbes will also vary with the individual host, including dramatic changes in the indigenous flora in hospitalized patients. Thus, only qualitative data (presence or absence of the organisms) are presented. Data for viruses are not listed because replication of viruses generally is associated with host tissue destruction or an immunologic response (although this can range from a clinically asymptomatic infection to host death).

Most diseases in humans are caused by infections with endogenous bacteria and yeasts or exposure to opportunistic molds, parasites, and viruses. However, some interactions between microbes and humans commonly lead to disease. The most common microbes responsible for human disease are summarized in this section. Arthropods, parasites in their own right, can also serve as vectors for human disease. A listing of the most common arthropod vectors and their associated diseases is included. Tables 2.2 and 2.3 are listings of fungi and parasites isolated from humans and their geographic distribution. For additional information about indigenous and pathogenic microbes, please consult the reference texts listed in the Bibliography.

Microbes of Humans

Microbes of Humans

Table 2.1 Human indigenous flora[a]

Organism	Prevalence of carriage in:[b]			
	Resp tract	**GI tract**	**GU tract**	**Skin, ear, and eye**
Abiotrophia adiacens	+	+	+	0
Abiotrophia defectiva	+	+	+	0
Acholeplasma laidlawii	+	0	0	0
Acidaminococcus fermentans	+	+	0	0
Acinetobacter spp.	+	+	+	+
Actinobacillus actinomycetemcomitans	+	0	0	0
Actinobacillus ureae	+	0	0	0
Actinomyces israelii	+	+	+	0
Actinomyces meyeri	+	+	+	0
Actinomyces naeslundii	+	+	+	0
Actinomyces odontolyticus	+	+	+	0
Actinomyces viscosus	+	+	+	0
Aerococcus viridans	0	0	0	+
Aeromonas spp.	0	+	0	0
Anuerorhabdus furcosus	0	+	0	0
Arcanobacterium haemolyticum	+	0	0	0
Arthrobacter agilis	0	0	0	+
Arthrobacter cumminsii	0	0	0	+

Bacillus spp.	o	+	o	+
Bacteroides caccae	o	+	o	o
Bacteroides capillosus	+	+	o	o
Bacteroides coagulans	o	+	+	o
Bacteroides distasonis	o	+	o	o
Bacteroides eggerthii	+	o	o	o
Bacteroides forsythus	o	+	o	o
Bacteroides fragilis	o	+	+	o
Bacteroides ovatus	+	o	o	o
Bacteroides pneumosintes	o	+	o	o
Bacteroides putredinis	o	+	o	o
Bacteroides thetaiotaomicron	o	+	o	o
Bacteroides vulgatus	+	+	+	o
Bacteroides, other spp.	o	+	o	o
Bifidobacterium adolescentis	o	+	o	o
Bifidobacterium angulatum	o	+	+	o
Bifidobacterium bifidum	o	+	+	o
Bifidobacterium breve	o	+	o	o
Bifidobacterium catenulatum	o	+	+	o
Bifidobacterium denitium	+	+	o	o
Bifidobacterium gallicum	o	+	o	o

(continued)

Microbes of Humans

Microbes of Humans

Table 2.1 Human indigenous flora[a] (continued)

Organism	Resp tract	GI tract	GU tract	Skin, ear, and eye
		Prevalence of carriage in:[b]		
Bifidobacterium infantis	0	+	0	0
Bifidobacterium longum	0	+	+	0
Bifidobacterium pseudocatenulatum	0	+	0	0
Bilophila wadsworthia	+	+	+	0
Blastocystis hominis	0	+	0	0
Blastoschizomyces capitatus	0	0	0	+
Brachyspira aalborgii	0	+	0	0
Brevibacterium epidermidis	0	0	0	+
Burkholderia cepacia	+	0	0	+
Butyrivibrio crossatus	0	+	0	0
Campylobacter concisus	+	0	0	0
Campylobacter curva	+	0	0	0
Campylobacter gracilis	+	0	0	0
Campylobacter recta	+	0	0	0
Campylobacter sputorum	+	+	0	0
Campylobacter ureolyticus	+	+	+	+
Candida albicans	+	+	+	+
Candida (Torulopsis) glabrata	+	+	+	0

Candida guilliermondii	+	+	0
Candida kefyr	+	+	0
Candida krusei	+	+	0
Candida parapsilosis	+	0	0
Candida tropicalis	+	+	0
Capnocytophaga spp.	+	0	0
Cardiobacterium hominis	0	+	0
Chilomastix mesnili	+	+	0
Chryseobacterium meningosepticum	0	0	0
Citrobacter spp.	0	+	+
Clostridium difficile	0	+	0
Clostridium perfringens	0	+	+
Clostridium, other spp.	0	+	+
Corynebacterium amycolatum	0	0	0
Corynebacterium auris	0	0	0
Corynebacterium durum	+	0	+
Corynebacterium glucuronolyticum	0	+	0
Corynebacterium jeikeium	0	0	+
Corynebacterium matruchotii	+	0	0
Corynebacterium minutissimum	0	0	+
Corynebacterium pseudodiphtheriticum	+	+	0

(continued)

Microbes of Humans

Microbes of Humans

Table 2.1 Human indigenous flora[a] *(continued)*

Organism	Prevalence of carriage in:[b]			
	Resp tract	GI tract	GU tract	Skin, ear, and eye
Corynebacterium striatum	0	0	0	+
Corynebacterium ulcerans	+	0	0	0
Corynebacterium xerosis	+	0	0	+
Cryptococcus albidus	+	0	0	0
Dermabacter hominis	0	0	0	+
Dermacoccus nishinomiyaensis	0	0	0	+
Desulfomonas pigra	0	+	0	0
Desulfovibrio spp.	0	+	0	0
Eikenella corrodens	+	+	+	0
Endolimax nana	0	+	0	0
Entamoeba coli	0	+	0	0
Entamoeba gingivalis	+	0	0	0
Entamoeba hartmanni	0	+	0	0
Entamoeba polecki	0	+	0	0
Enterobacter spp.	+	+	0	0
Enterococcus spp.	0	+	+	0
Enteromonas hominis	0	+	0	0
Epidermophyton floccosum	0	0	0	+

Escherichia coli	0	+	0
Eubacterium spp.	+	+	+
Fusobacterium alocis	+	0	0
Fusobacterium gonidiaformans	0	+	+
Fusobacterium mortiferum	0	+	0
Fusobacterium naviforme	0	+	+
Fusobacterium necrogenes	+	+	0
Fusobacterium necrophorum	+	+	0
Fusobacterium nucleatum	0	0	+
Fusobacterium perfoetens	+	+	0
Fusobacterium periodonticum	+	0	0
Fusobacterium russii	0	+	0
Fusobacterium varium	0	+	+
Gardnerella vaginalis	0	0	0
Gemella haemolysans	+	0	0
Gemella morbillorum	+	+	0
Haemophilus aphrophilus	+	0	0
Haemophilus haemolyticus	+	0	0
Haemophilus influenzae	+	+	+
Haemophilus parahaemolyticus	+	0	0
Haemophilus parainfluenzae	+	+	+

(continued)

Microbes of Humans

Microbes of Humans

Table 2.1 Human indigenous flora[a] *(continued)*

Organism	Prevalence of carriage in:[b]			
	Resp tract	GI tract	GU tract	Skin, ear, and eye
Haemophilus paraphrophilus	+	+	0	0
Haemophilus segnis	+	+	0	0
Hafnia alvei	+	+	0	0
Helcococcus kunzii	0	0	0	+
Helicobacter cinaedi	0	+	0	0
Helicobacter fennelliae	0	+	0	0
Helicobacter pylori	+	+	0	0
Iodamoeba butschlii	0	+	0	0
Kingella denitrificans	+	0	0	0
Kingella kingae	+	0	0	0
Klebsiella spp.	+	+	0	0
Kocuria kristinae	0	0	0	+
Kocuria rosea	0	0	0	+
Kocuria varians	0	0	0	+
Kytococcus sedentarius	0	0	0	+
Lactobacillus acidophilus	+	+	+	0
Lactobacillus breve	+	0	0	0
Lactobacillus casei	+	0	+	0

Lactobacillus cellobiosus	0	0		0
Lactobacillus fermentum	+	+	+	0
Lactobacillus reuteri	0	+	+	0
Lactobacillus salivarius	+	+	0	0
Lactococcus garvieae	0	0	+	0
Leptotrichia buccalis	+	+	+	0
Listeria monocytogenes	0	+	0	0
Malassezia furfur	0	0	0	+
Malassezia sympodialis	0	0	0	+
Megasphaera elsdenii	+	+	0	0
Micrococcus luteus/lylae	0	0	0	+
Microsporum audouinii	0	0	0	+
Microsporum ferrugineum	0	0	+	+
Miksuokella multiacidus	0	+	+	0
Mobiluncus curtisii	0	+	+	0
Mobiluncus mulieris	0	0	+	0
Moraxella atlantae	+	0	0	0
Moraxella catarrhalis	+	0	0	0
Moraxella lacunata	+	0	0	0
Moraxella nonliquefaciens	+	0	0	0
Moraxella osloensis	+	0	0	0

(continued)

Microbes of Humans

Microbes of Humans

Table 2.1 Human indigenous flora[a] (continued)

Organism	Prevalence of carriage in:[b]			
	Resp tract	GI tract	GU tract	Skin, ear, and eye
Morganella morganii	0	+	0	0
Mycoplasma buccale	+	0	0	0
Mycoplasma fermentans	+	0	+	0
Mycoplasma genitalium	0	0	+	0
Mycoplasma hominis	0	0	+	0
Mycoplasma lipophilum	+	0	0	0
Mycoplasma orale	+	0	0	0
Mycoplasma penetrans	0	0	+	0
Mycoplasma salivarium	+	0	0	0
Neisseria cinerea	+	0	0	0
Neisseria flavescens	+	0	0	0
Neisseria lactamica	+	0	0	0
Neisseria meningitidis	+	0	+	0
Neisseria mucosa	+	0	0	0
Neisseria polysaccharea	+	0	0	0
Neisseria sicca	+	0	0	0
Neisseria subflava	+	0	0	0
Oligella ureolytica	0	0	+	0

Oligella urethralis	0	0	+	0
Pasteurella multocida	+	0	0	0
Peptostreptococcus spp.	+	+	+	+
Porphyromonas asaccharolytica	+	+	+	0
Porphyromonas endodontalis	+	0	0	0
Porphyromonas gingivalis	+	+	+	0
Porphyromonas, other spp.	+	0	+	0
Prevotella bivia	0	0	0	0
Prevotella buccae	+	0	0	0
Prevotella buccalis	+	0	0	0
Prevotella corporis	+	0	+	0
Prevotella denticola	+	0	0	0
Prevotella disiens	+	0	+	0
Prevotella intermedia	+	0	0	0
Prevotella loescheii	+	0	0	0
Prevotella melaninogenica	+	0	0	0
Prevotella nigrescens	+	0	0	0
Prevotella oris	+	0	0	0
Prevotella, other spp.	+	+	+	+
Propionibacterium acnes	0	0	0	+
Propionibacterium avidum	0	0	0	+

(continued)

Microbes of Humans

Table 2.1 Human indigenous flora[a] (continued)

Organism	Prevalence of carriage in:[b]			
	Resp tract	GI tract	GU tract	Skin, ear, and eye
Propionibacterium granulosum	0	0	0	+
Propionibacterium propionicus	+	0	0	0
Propioniferax innocuum	0	0	0	+
Proteus spp.	0	+	+	0
Providencia spp.	0	+	+	0
Pseudomonas aeruginosa	+	+	0	0
Pseudomonas, other spp.	0	+	0	0
Psychrobacter phenylpyruvica	+	0	0	0
Retortamonas intestinalis	0	+	0	0
Rhodotorula spp.	0	0	0	+
Rothia dentocariosa	+	0	0	0
Ruminococcus spp.	0	+	0	0
Selenomonas spp.	+	+	0	0
Serpulina spp.	0	+	0	0
Staphylococcus aureus	+	+	+	+
Staphylococcus, coagulase negative	+	+	+	+
Stomatococcus mucilaginosus	+	0	0	0
Streptococcus agalactiae	+	+	+	0

Streptococcus bovis	0	+	0	0
Streptococcus pneumoniae	+	0	0	0
Streptococcus pyogenes	+	+	+	+
Streptococcus, group C,F, or G	+	+	+	0
Streptococcus, viridans group	+	+	+	0
Succinivibrio dextrinosolvens	0	+	0	0
Tissierella praeacuta	0	+	0	0
Treponema denticola	+	0	+	0
Treponema minutum	0	0	0	0
Treponema pectinovorum	+	0	+	0
Treponema phagedenis	0	0	+	0
Treponema refringens	0	0	0	0
Treponema skiliodontium	+	0	0	0
Treponema socranskii	+	0	0	0
Treponema vincentii	+	+	0	0
Trichomonas hominis	0	0	0	0
Trichomonas tenax	+	0	0	0
Trichophyton concentricum	0	0	0	+
Trichophyton gourvilii	0	0	0	+
Trichophyton kanei	0	0	0	+
Trichophyton megninii	0	0	0	+

(continued)

Microbes of Humans

Microbes of Humans

Table 2.1 Human indigenous flora[a] (*continued*)

Organism	Prevalence of carriage in:[b]			
	Resp tract	GI tract	GU tract	Skin, ear, and eye
Trichophyton mentagrophytes	0	0	0	+
Trichophyton raubitschekii	0	0	0	+
Trichophyton rubrum	0	0	0	+
Trichophyton schoenleinii	0	0	0	+
Trichophyton soudanense	0	0	0	+
Trichophyton tonsurans	0	0	0	+
Trichophyton violaceum	0	0	0	+
Trichophyton yaoundei	0	0	0	+
Turicella otitidis	0	0	0	+
Ureaplasma urealyticum	0	0	+	0
Veillonella atypica	+	0	0	0
Veillonella dispar	+	0	0	0
Veillonella parvula	+	+	0	0
Weeksella virosa	0	0	+	0
Yersinia frederiksenii	0	+	0	0
Yersinia kristensenii	0	+	0	0

[a] Adapted from P. R. Murray, Human microbiota, p. 295–306, *in* L. Collier, A. Balows, and M. Sussman (ed.), *Topley & Wilson's Microbiology and Microbial Infections*, 9th ed., Arnold, London, 1998.
[b] Resp, respiratory; GI, gastrointestinal; GU, genitourinary; +, commonly present; 0, not typically isolated in healthy individuals.

Microbes Responsible for Human Disease[a]

UPPER RESPIRATORY INFECTIONS
Pharyngitis
Bacteria
- *Streptococcus*, group A
- *Streptococcus*, group C
- *Archanobacterium haemolyticum*
- *Chlamydia pneumoniae*
- *Neisseria gonorrhoeae*
- *Corynebacterium diphtheriae*
- *Corynebacterium ulcerans*
- *Mycoplasma pneumoniae*

Viruses
- Respiratory syncytial virus
- Rhinovirus
- Coronavirus
- Adenovirus
- HSV
- Parainfluenza virus
- Influenza virus
- Coxsackievirus groups A and B
- EBV
- CMV
- Human immunodeficiency virus

Sinusitis
Bacteria
- *Streptococcus pneumoniae*
- *Haemophilus influenzae*
- Mixed anaerobes
- *Staphylococcus aureus*
- *Moraxella catarrhalis*
- *Streptococcus*, group A
- *Chlamydia pneumoniae*
- *Pseudomonas aeruginosa* (and other gram-negative bacilli)

Viruses
- Rhinovirus
- Influenza virus
- Parainfluenza virus
- Adenovirus

Fungi
- *Aspergillus* (allergic sinusitis)

Hyphomycetes (allergic sinusitis)
Zygomycetes (invasive disease)

EAR INFECTIONS
Otitis externa
Bacteria
  Pseudomonas aeruginosa (swimmer's ear; malignant
    otitis)
  Staphylococcus aureus (pustule)
  Streptococcus, group A (erysipelas)
Fungi
  Aspergillus spp.
  Candida albicans
Otitis media
Bacteria
  Streptococcus pneumoniae
  Haemophilus influenzae
  Moraxella catarrhalis
  Staphylococcus aureus
  Streptococcus, group A
  Mixed anaerobes
Viruses
  Respiratory syncytial virus
  Influenza virus
  Enterovirus
  Rhinovirus

PLEUROPULMONARY AND BRONCHIAL INFECTIONS
Bronchitis
Bacteria
  Bordetella pertussis
  Mycoplasma pneumoniae
  Chlamydia pneumoniae
  Moraxella catarrhalis
  Haemophilus influenzae
  Streptococcus pneumoniae
Viruses
  Influenza virus
  Rhinovirus
  Respiratory syncytial virus
  Parainfluenza virus
  Adenovirus

Coronavirus
Coxsackievirus group A

Empyema
Bacteria
Staphylococcus aureus
Streptococcus pneumoniae
Streptococcus, group A
Bacteroides fragilis
Klebsiella pneumoniae (and other gram-negative bacilli)
Actinomyces spp.
Nocardia spp.
Mycobacterium tuberculosis (and other myco-bacterial spp.)
Fungi
Aspergillus spp.
Pneumocystis carinii
Parasites
Entamoeba histolytica

Pneumonia
Bacteria
Streptococcus pneumoniae
Staphylococcus aureus
Haemophilus influenzae
Neisseria meningitidis
Mycoplasma pneumoniae
Chlamydia spp. (*C. trachomatis*, *C. pneumoniae*, *C. psittaci*)
Klebsiella pneumoniae (and other *Enterobacteriaceae*)
Pseudomonas aeruginosa
Burkholderia pseudomallei
Legionella pneumophila (and other *Legionella* spp.)
Francisella tularensis
Bacteroides fragilis (and other anaerobes in mixed infections)
Nocardia spp.
Rhodococcus equi
Mycobacterium tuberculosis (and other *Mycobacterium* spp.)
Coxiella burnetii
Rickettsia rickettsii
Many other bacteria

Viruses
    Respiratory syncytial virus
    Parainfluenza viruses
    Influenza viruses
    Adenovirus
    Rhinovirus
    Enteroviruses (rhinovirus, coxsackieviruses, poliovirus)
    Herpesviruses (CMV, EBV, VZV, HSV)
Fungi
    Pneumocystis carinii
    Cryptococcus neoformans
    Histoplasma capsulatum
    Blastomyces dermatitidis
    Coccidioides immitis
    Paracoccidioides brasiliensis
    Aspergillus spp.
    Phycomyces spp.
Parasites
    Ascaris lumbricoides
    Strongyloides stercoralis
    Toxoplasma gondii
    Paragonimus westermani

URINARY TRACT INFECTIONS
Cystitis and pyelonephritis
Bacteria
    Escherichia coli
    Proteus mirabilis
    Klebsiella spp.
    Enterobacter spp.
    Salmonella typhi
    Pseudomonas aeruginosa
    Staphylococcus aureus (primarily hematogenous source)
    Staphylococcus saprophyticus (primarily in young adult women)
    Staphylococcus, other spp. (primarily catheter-associated)
    Streptococcus, group B
    Enterococcus spp.
    Aerococcus urinae
    Mycobacterium tuberculosis (hematogenous source)

Viruses
   Adenovirus (hemorrhagic cystitis)
Fungi
   Candida albicans
   Candida glabrata
   Candida, other spp.
Parasites
   Schistosoma haematobium
Renal calculi
Bacteria
   Proteus spp.
   Morganella morganii
   Klebsiella pneumoniae
   Corynebacterium urealyticum
   Staphylococcus saprophyticus
   Ureaplasma urealyticum
Prostatitis
Bacteria
   Escherichia coli
   Klebsiella spp.
   Proteus mirabilis
   Enterobacter spp.
   Enterococcus spp.
   Neisseria gonorrhoeae
   Mycobacterium tuberculosis (and other myco-
      bacterial spp.)
Fungi
   Candida spp.
   Cryptococcus neoformans

INTRA-ABDOMINAL INFECTIONS
Peritonitis
Bacteria
   Escherichia coli
   Klebsiella pneumoniae (and other gram-negative
      enteric bacilli)
   Pseudomonas aeruginosa
   Streptococcus pneumoniae
   Staphylococcus aureus
   Enterococcus spp.
   Bacteroides fragilis group
   Bacteroides, other spp.
   Fusobacterium spp.

      Clostridium spp.

      Peptostreptococcus spp.

      Neisseria gonorrhoeae (perihepatitis, Fitz-Hugh and
        Curtis syndrome)

      Chlamydia trachomatis (Fitz-Hugh and Curtis
        syndrome)

      Mycobacterium tuberculosis

   Fungi

      Candida albicans (and other *Candida* spp.)

   Parasites

      Strongyloides stercoralis

Dialysis-associated peritonitis

   Bacteria

      Staphylococcus, coagulase-negative spp.

      Staphylococcus aureus

      Streptococcus spp.

      Corynebacterium spp.

      Propionibacterium spp.

      Escherichia coli (and other gram-negative enteric
        bacilli)

      Pseudomonas aeruginosa

      Acinetobacter spp.

   Fungi

      Candida albicans

      Candida parapsilosis (and other *Candida* spp.)

      Aspergillus spp.

      Fusarium spp.

Visceral abscesses

   Bacteria

      Escherichia coli (and other gram-negative enteric
        bacilli)

      Enterococcus spp.

      Staphylococcus aureus

      Bacteroides fragilis group

      Fusobacterium spp.

      Actinomyces spp.

      Aerobic and anaerobic polymicrobic infections

      Yersinia enterocolitica

      Mycobacterium tuberculosis

      Mycobacterium avium complex (and other myco-
        bacterial spp.)

   Fungi

      Candida albicans (and other *Candida* spp.)

Microbes of Humans

Parasites
    Entamoeba histolytica (primarily hepatic abscesses)
    Echinococcus (hepatic abscesses)

CARDIOVASCULAR INFECTIONS
Endocarditis
Bacteria
    Streptococcus, viridans group (primarily *S. mutans*,
       S. sanguis)
    Streptococcus bovis
    Streptococcus pneumoniae
    Abiotrophia spp. (*A. adiacens*, *A. defectiva*)
    Staphylococcus aureus
    Staphylococcus, coagulase-negative
    Stomatococcus mucilaginosus
    Enterococcus spp. (primarily *E. faecalis*, *E. faecium*)
    Haemophilus spp. (HACEK; primarily *H. aphrophilus*,
       H. paraphrophilus, *H. parainfluenzae*)
    Actinobacillus actinomycetemcomitans (HACEK)
    Cardiobacterium hominis (HACEK)
    Eikenella corrodens (HACEK)
    Kingella spp. (HACEK; primarily *K. kingae*)
    Salmonella spp.
    Serratia spp. (and other enteric gram-negative bacilli)
    Pseudomonas aeruginosa
    Brucella spp.
    Bartonella spp. (primarily *B. henselae*)
    Corynebacterium spp. (primarily in damaged or
       prosthetic valves)
    Erysipelothrix rhusiopathiae
    Coxiella burnetii
    Chlamydia psittaci
Fungi
    Candida spp. (*C. parapsilosis*, *C. albicans*,
       C. tropicalis, other spp.)
    Aspergillus spp.
Myocarditis
Bacteria
    Corynebacterium diphtheriae
    Clostridium perfringens
    Streptococcus, group A
    Borrelia burgdorferi
    Neisseria meningitidis

       Staphylococcus aureus
       Mycoplasma pneumoniae
       Chlamydia spp. (*C. pneumoniae, C. psittaci*)
       Rickettsia spp. (*R. rickettsii, R. tsutsugamushi*)

Viruses
    Coxsackievirus groups A and B
    Echoviruses
    Poliovirus
    Mumps virus
    Rubeola virus
    Influenza virus A and B
    Herpesviruses (VZV, CMV, EBV)
    Adenovirus
    Flaviviruses
    Arenaviruses

Fungi
    Aspergillus spp.
    Candida spp.
    Cryptococcus neoformans

Parasites
    Trypanosoma spp.
    Trichinella spiralis
    Toxoplasma gondii

Pericarditis

Bacteria
    Streptococcus pneumoniae
    Staphylococcus aureus
    Neisseria spp. (*N. meningitidis, N. gonorrhoeae*)
    Mycoplasma pneumoniae
    Mycobacterium tuberculosis
    Mycobacterium (other spp.)

Viruses
    Coxsackievirus groups A and B
    Echovirus
    Adenovirus
    Mumps virus
    Influenza virus
    Herpesviruses (EBV, VZV, CMV, HSV)

Fungi
    Histoplasma capsulatum
    Coccidioides immitis
    Blastomyces dermatitidis
    Cryptococcus neoformans

    Candida spp.
    Aspergillus spp.
Parasites
    Toxoplasma gondii
    Entamoeba histolytica
    Schistosoma spp.

SEPSIS
Transfusion-associated sepsis
Bacteria
    Yersinia enterocolitica
    Staphylococcus, coagulase-negative spp.
    Staphylococcus aureus
    Pseudomonas fluorescens
    Pseudomonas putida
    Salmonella spp.
    Serratia marcescens (and other *Enterobacteriaceae*)
    Campylobacter jejuni
    Treponema pallidum
    Bacillus cereus (and other *Bacillus* spp.)
    Borrelia spp. (agents responsible for relapsing
       fever)
Viruses
    Hepatitis virus (A, B, C, D)
    CMV
    EBV
    Human immunodeficiency virus
    Human T-cell leukemia virus
    Parvovirus B19
    Colorado tick fever virus
Parasites
    Plasmodium spp.
    Babesia microti
    Toxoplasma gondii
    Trypanosoma cruzi
    Leishmania spp.

CENTRAL NERVOUS SYSTEM INFECTIONS
Meningitis
Bacteria
    Escherichia coli
    Streptococcus, group B
    Streptococcus pneumoniae

Neisseria meningitidis

Listeria monocytogenes

Haemophilus influenzae (typeable and nontypeable strains)

Other gram-negative bacilli (associated with sepsis, neurosurgery, or shunts)

Staphylococcus spp. (associated with neurosurgery or shunts)

Propionibacterium spp. (associated with neuro-surgery or shunts)

Nocardia spp.

Treponema pallidum

Brucella spp.

Borrelia burgdorferi

Leptospira spp.

Mycobacterium tuberculosis

Mycobacterium avium complex (and other spp.)

Viruses

Enteroviruses (echovirus, coxsackievirus groups A and B, poliovirus)

Flaviviruses

Orbivirus (Colorado tick fever)

Mumps virus

HSV

Human immunodeficiency virus

Fungi

Cryptococcus neoformans

Histoplasma capsulatum

Coccidioides immitis

Candida spp.

Parasites

Naegleria fowleri

Acanthamoeba spp.

Angiostrongylus cantonensis

Encephalitis

Bacteria

Listeria monocytogenes

Treponema pallidum

Leptospira spp.

Actinomyces spp.

Nocardia spp.

Borrelia spp. (associated with Lyme disease and relapsing fever)

    Rickettsia rickettsii
    Coxiella burnetii
    Mycoplasma pneumoniae
    Mycobacterium tuberculosis
Viruses
    Enteroviruses (poliovirus, coxsackievirus, echovirus,
        hepatitis A virus)
    Herpesviruses (HSV, VZV, EBV, CMV)
    Alphaviruses (EEE, WEE, VEE)
    Flaviviruses (SLE, Japanese encephalitis, dengue,
        Murray Valley encephalitis)
    Bunyaviruses (La Crosse virus, Rift Valley virus)
    Arenaviruses (lymphocytic choriomeningitis virus,
        Machupo virus, Lassa virus, Junin virus)
    Filoviruses (Ebola virus, Marburg virus)
    Rabies virus
    Human immunodeficiency virus
    Mumps virus
    Measles virus
    Rubella virus
    Adenovirus
Fungi
    Cryptococcus neoformans
    Histoplasma capsulatum
Parasites
    Naegleria fowleri
    Acanthamoeba spp.
    Toxoplasma gondii
    Plasmodium falciparum
    Trypanosoma spp.

Brain abscess
Bacteria
    Staphylococcus aureus
    Enterobacteriaceae (*Proteus*, *Escherichia*, *Klebsiella*,
        and others)
    Pseudomonas aeruginosa
    Streptococcus, viridans group (*S. anginosus*,
        S. intermedium, *S. constellatus*, and other spp.)
    Bacteroides spp.
    Prevotella spp.
    Porphyromonas spp.
    Fusobacterium spp.
    Peptostreptococcus spp.

Microbes of Humans

Actinomyces spp.
Clostridium spp. (associated with neurosurgery)
Listeria monocytogenes
Nocardia spp.
Rhodococcus equi
Mycobacterium tuberculosis
Fungi
Cryptococcus neoformans
Candida spp.
Coccidioides immitis
Aspergillus spp.
Parasites
Acanthamoeba spp.
Toxoplasma gondii

SKIN AND SOFT TISSUE INFECTIONS
Bacteria
Staphylococcus aureus
Staphylococcus, coagulase-negative (associated with foreign bodies)
Streptococcus, group A (other β-hemolytic species less commonly)
Pseudomonas aeruginosa
Enterobacteriaceae (usually in mixed wound infections)
Vibrio vulnificus (other *Vibrio* spp. less commonly)
Bacteroides fragilis (usually in mixed infections)
Clostridium perfringens (and other *Clostridium* spp.)
Bacillus anthracis
Francisella tularensis
Pasteurella multocida (animal bite wounds)
Eikenella corrodens (human bite wounds)
Bartonella spp. (*B. henselae*, *B. quintana*)
Erysipelothrix rhusiopathiae
Corynebacterium minutissimum (cause of erythrasma)
Treponema pallidum
Nocardia spp. (particularly *N. brasiliensis*)
Mycobacterium spp. (particularly *M. marinum*, *M. ulcerans*, rapid-growers)
Viruses
Many viruses with skin manifestations (rashes, erythema, papules, vesicles, pustules)
Fungi
Candida albicans (and other *Candida* spp.)

Aspergillus spp.
Blastomyces dermatitidis
Dermatophytes
Many fungi responsible for chromomycosis and
mycetoma
Parasites
Onchocerca volvulus
Mansonella streptocerca
Leishmania spp.

GASTROINTESTINAL INFECTIONS

Bacteria
Salmonella spp.
Shigella spp.
Campylobacter spp. (*C. jejuni*, *C. coli*, other spp.)
Vibrio spp. (*V. cholerae*, *V. parahaemolyticus*, other spp.)
Yersinia enterocolitica
Escherichia coli (ETEC, EIEC, EHEC, EPEC, EAggEC)
Edwardsiella tarda
Staphylococcus aureus (intoxication)
Bacillus cereus (intoxication)
Pseudomonas aeruginosa
Aeromonas spp. (*A. hydrophila*, *A. caviae*, *A. veronii*, other spp.)
Plesiomonas shigelloides
Bacteroides fragilis
Clostridium botulinum (intoxication)
Clostridium perfringens
Clostridium difficile
Viruses
Rotavirus (primarily group A)
Caliciviruses (including Norwalk virus and Norwalk-like viruses)
Astrovirus
Adenovirus (primarily types 40 and 41)
Coronavirus
CMV
Torovirus
Parasites
Giardia lamblia
Entamoeba histolytica

> *Balantidium coli*
> *Cryptosporidium parvum*
> *Isospora belli*
> Microsporidia
> *Cyclospora cayetanensis*
> *Diphyllobothrium latum*
> *Anisakis* spp.
> *Trichinella spiralis*
> *Strongyloides stercoralis*

BONE AND JOINT INFECTIONS
Osteomyelitis
Bacteria
> *Staphylococcus aureus*
> *Staphylococcus*, coagulase-negative (associated with foreign body)
> *Streptococcus*, β-hemolytic groups
> *Streptococcus pneumoniae*
> *Escherichia coli*
> *Salmonella* spp. (and other *Enterobacteriaceae*)
> *Pseudomonas aeruginosa*
> *Mycobacterium tuberculosis* (and other *Mycobacterium* spp.)
> Many other species can infrequently cause disease

Fungi
> *Candida* spp.
> *Aspergillus* spp.
> *Cryptococcus neoformans*
> *Blastomyces dermatitidis*
> *Coccidiodes immitis*

Arthritis
Bacteria
> *Staphylococcus aureus*
> *Neisseria gonorrhoeae*
> *Streptococcus pneumoniae*
> *Salmonella* spp.
> *Pasteurella multocida*
> *Mycobacterium* spp.

Viruses
> Rubella virus
> Hepatitis B virus
> Mumps virus
> Lymphocytic choriomeningitis virus

Parvovirus B19
Human immunodeficiency virus
Fungi
   Sporothrix schenckii
   Coccidioides immitis
   Candida albicans (and other *Candida* spp.)

GENITAL INFECTIONS
Genital ulcers
Bacteria
   Treponema pallidum
   Haemophilus ducreyi
   Chlamydia trachomatis (lymphogranuloma
      venereum)
   Francisella tularensis
   Calymmatobacterium granulomatis (granuloma
      inguinale)
   Mycobacterium tuberculosis
Viruses
   HSV
Fungi
   Histoplasma capsulatum
Urethritis
Bacteria
   Neisseria gonorrhoeae
   Chlamydia trachomatis
   Ureaplasma urealyticum
Vaginitis
Bacteria
   Mobiluncus spp.
   Gardnerella vaginalis
   Mycoplasma hominis
Fungi
   Candida spp.
Parasites
   Trichomonas vaginalis
Cervicitis
Bacteria
   Neisseria gonorrhoeae
   Neisseria meningitidis
   Chlamydia trachomatis
   Streptococcus, group B
   Mycobacterium tuberculosis

Microbes of Humans

Actinomyces spp. (associated with use of intrauterine devices)

Viruses
  HSV
  CMV
  Adenovirus
  Measles virus
  Papillomavirus
Parasites
  Enterobius vermicularis

EYE INFECTIONS
Conjunctivitis
Bacteria
  Streptococcus pneumoniae
  Streptococcus, group B
  Streptococcus, viridans group
  Staphylococcus aureus (and other spp.)
  Moraxella catarrhalis (and other spp.)
  Haemophilus aegyptius
  Haemophilus ducreyi
  Neisseria gonorrhoeae (and other spp.)
  Pseudomonas aeruginosa
  Corynebacterium diphtheriae
  Francisella tularensis
  Borrelia burgdorferi
  Bartonella henselae
  Chlamydia trachomatis
Viruses
  Adenovirus (keratoconjunctivitis; hemorrhagic conjunctivitis)
  Herpesviruses (HSV, VZV, EBV)
  Papillomavirus
  Rubella virus
  Influenza virus
  Measles virus
Fungi
  Candida spp.
  Sporothrix schenckii
Parasites
  Onchocerca volvulus
  Loa loa
  Wuchereria bancrofti

Leishmania donovani
Microsporidia, most commonly *Encephalitozoon* spp.
Toxocara canis

Keratitis

Bacteria

Staphylococcus aureus (and other *Staphylococcus* spp.)
Streptococcus pneumoniae
Streptococcus, viridans group
Streptococcus, group A
Enterococcus faecalis
Pseudomonas aeruginosa
Proteus mirabilis (and other enteric gram-negative bacilli)
Bacillus spp. (associated with penetrating eye injury)
Clostridium perfringens
Neisseria gonorrhoeae
Many other bacteria are rare causes of keratitis

Viruses

Herpesviruses (HSV, VZV, EBV)
Adenovirus
Measles virus

Fungi

Fusarium solani
Aspergillus spp.
Candida spp.
Many other fungi (particularly septated filamentous fungi) involved

Parasites

Onchocerca volvulus
Acanthamoeba spp.
Leishmania braziliensis
Trypanosoma spp.
Microsporidia (*Nosema* spp., *Encephalitozoon* spp.)

Endophthalmitis

Bacteria

Staphylococcus aureus (and other *Staphylococcus* spp.)
Pseudomonas aeruginosa
Propionibacterium spp.
Corynebacterium spp.
Bacillus spp. (after penetrating eye injury)
Many other bacteria are rare causes of endophthalmitis

Viruses
  Herpesviruses (HSV, CMV, VZV)
  Rubella virus
  Measles virus
Fungi
  Candida albicans (and other spp.)
  Aspergillus spp.
  Histoplasma capsulatum
  Opportunistic fungi following penetrating eye injury
Parasites
  Toxoplasma gondii
  Toxocara spp.
  Cysticercus cellulosae

GRANULOMATOUS INFECTIONS
Bacteria
  Brucella spp.
  Francisella tularensis
  Listeria monocytogenes
  Burkholderia pseudomallei
  Actinomyces spp.
  Bartonella henselae
  Tropheryma whippelii
  Mycobacterium spp.
  Chlamydia trachomatis
  Coxiella burnetii
  Treponema pallidum
  Treponema carateum
  Nocardia spp.
Viruses
  CMV
  Measles virus
  Mumps virus
  EBV
Fungi
  Cryptococcus neoformans
  Candida spp.
  Sporothrix schenckii
  Histoplasma capsulatum
  Paracoccidioides brasiliensis
  Coccidioides immitis
  Blastomyces dermatitidis
  Aspergillus spp.

Phialophora spp.
Pseudallescheria boydii
Parasites
    Leishmania spp.
    Toxoplasma gondii
    Schistosoma spp.
    Toxocara spp

[a]HSV, herpes simplex virus; CMV, cytomegalovirus; EBV, Epstein-Barr virus; VZV, varicella-zoster virus; HACEK, *Haemophilus–Actinobacillus–Cardiobacterium–Eikenella–Kingella;* EEE, Eastern equine encephalitis; WEE, Western equine encephalitis; VEE, Venezualan equine encephalitis; SLE, St. Louis encephalitis; ETEC, enterotoxigenic *E. coli;* EIEC, enteroinvasive *E. coli;* EHEC, enterohemorrhagic *E. coli;* EPEC, enteropathogenic *E. coli;* EAggEC, enteraggregative *E. coli.*

Arthropod Vectors of Medically Important Diseases

Arachnida
  Acari (ticks)

Amblyomma	*Ehrlichia chaffeensis* (human monocytic ehrlichiosis)
	Francisella tularensis (tularemia)
	Rickettsia rickettsii (Rocky Mountain spotted fever)
Dermacentor	*Francisella tularensis* (tularemia)
	Rickettsia rickettsii (Rocky Mountain spotted fever)
	Coltivirus (Colorado tick fever)
Ixodes	*Babesia* spp. (babesiosis)
	Borrelia burgdorferi (Lyme disease)
	Borrelia spp. (relapsing fever)
	Ehrlichia phagocytophila-equi group (human granulocytic ehrlichiosis)
Ornithodoros	*Borrelia* spp. (relapsing fever)
Rhipicephalus	*Ehrlichia canis* (ehrlichiosis)
	Rickettsia conorii (boutonneuse fever)

Rickettsia rickettsii (Rocky Mountain spotted fever)

Acari (mites)
    Leptotrombidium   *Orientia* (*Rickettsia*) *tsutsugamushi* (scrub typhus)
    Liponyssoides   *Rickettsia akari* (rickettsialpox)

Crustacea
    Copepoda (copepods)   *Diphyllobothrium* (diphyllobothriasis)
    Dracunculus (Guinea worm disease)
    Gnathostoma (Gnathostomiasis)
    Decapods   *Paragonimus* (paragonimiasis)
    (crabs, crayfish)

Insecta
    Anopleura (lice)
    Pediculus   *Borrelia recurrentis* (epidemic relapsing fever)
    Bartonella quintana (trench fever)
    Pediculus capitis (head louse)
    Pediculus humanus (body louse)
    Rickettsia prowazekii (epidemic typhus)
    Phthirus   *Phthirus pubis* (pubic louse)
    Diptera (mosquitos, flies)
    Aedes   Flavivirus (dengue, yellow fever)
    Other arboviruses (encephalitis)
    Anopheles   Arboviruses (encephalitis)
    Brugia malayi (filariasis)
    Plasmodium spp. (malaria)
    Chrysops   *Francisella tularensis* (tularemia)
    Loa loa (loiasis)
    Culex   Arboviruses (encephalitis)
    Brugia spp. (filariasis)

Microbes of Humans

	Wuchereria spp. (filariasis)
Culicoides	*Mansonella* spp. (filariasis)
Glossina	*Trypanosoma brucei* (African sleeping sickness)
Phlebotomus, Lutzomyia	*Bartonella bacilliformis* (bartonellosis)
	Leishmania spp. (leishmaniasis)
	Phlebovirus (sandfly fever)
Simulium	*Mansonella ozzardi* (filariasis)
	Onchocerca volvulus (onchocerciasis)
Hemiptera (bed bugs, kissing bugs)	
Panstrongylus, Rhodnius, Triatoma	*Trypanosoma cruzi* (Chagas' disease)
Siphonaptera (fleas)	
Ctenocephalides spp.	*Dipylidium caninum* (dog tapeworm disease)
Nosopsyllus spp.	*Rickettsia typhi* (murine typhus)
Xenopsylla spp.	*Rickettsia typhi* (murine typhus)
	Yersinia pestis (plague)

Microbes of Humans

Microbes of Humans

Table 2.2 Fungal pathogens and geographic distribution

Fungi	Human body sites	Geographic distribution
Yeasts		
Candida spp.	Opportunistic pathogen involving any part of body	Worldwide
Cryptococcus neoformans	Opportunistic pathogen primarily involving lungs and central nervous system; other body sites can be infected	Worldwide
Cryptococcus, other spp.	Opportunistic pathogen rarely implicated in disease	Worldwide
Blastoschizomyces capitatus	Opportunistic pathogen uncommonly implicated in systemic infections	Worldwide
Geotrichum candidum	Opportunistic pathogen uncommonly implicated in systemic infections	Worldwide
Hansenula spp.	Opportunistic pathogen uncommonly implicated in systemic infections	Worldwide
Malassezia furfur	Opportunistic pathogen involving skin surface (tinea versicolor) and systemic disease (associated with lipid therapy)	Worldwide

Rhodotorula spp.	Opportunistic pathogen uncommonly implicated in systemic infections	Worldwide
Trichosporon spp.	Opportunistic pathogen involving skin surface (white piedra); systemic infections in immunocompromised patients	Worldwide
Pneumocystis carinii	Opportunistic pathogen primarily involving respiratory tract	Worldwide
Dimorphic fungi		
Blastomyces dermatitidis	Blastomycosis is primarily a pulmonary infection with dissemination to skin, genitourinary tract, bone, and central nervous system	Ohio and Mississippi River valleys, as well as Missouri and Arkansas River basins; southern Canada, and portions of Africa
Coccidioides immitis	Coccidioidomycosis is primarily a pulmonary infection with dissemination to skin, bone, joints, lymph nodes, adrenal glands, and central nervous system	Southwestern U.S., northwestern Mexico, Argentina, and other dry areas of Central and South America

(continued)

Microbes of Humans

Microbes of Humans

Table 2.2 Fungal pathogens and geographic distribution *(continued)*

Fungi	Human body sites	Geographic distribution
Histoplasma capsulatum	Histoplasmosis is primarily a pulmonary infection with dissemination to central nervous system, adrenal glands, mucocutaneous surfaces, and other tissues	Temperate, tropical, and subtropical regions throughout the world, particularly Ohio, Missouri, and Mississippi River valleys, southern portions of Canada, and areas in Central and South America
H. capsulatum, var. *duboisii*	African histoplasmosis; pulmonary infection less common with more frequent involvement of skin and bones	Central Africa (between 20°N and 20°S)
Paracoccidioides brasiliensis	Paracoccidioidomycosis (South American blastomycosis) is primarily a pulmonary infection with dissemination commonly to nose and mouth, less commonly to lymph nodes, spleen, liver, gastrointestinal tract, and adrenal glands	Central and South America
Penicillium marneffei	Disseminated infection involving bone, skin, lung, lymph nodes, genitourinary and gastrointestinal tracts, central nervous system, and other tissues	Mountainous provinces of northern Thailand, Laos, Myanmar, and southeastern China

Sporothrix schenckii	Sporotrichosis involving skin and subcutaneous tissues with dissemination commonly via lymphatics to lymph nodes and, less commonly, to other internal organs	Worldwide, primarily in soil and decaying plant material
Cutaneous fungi		
Epidermophyton floccosum	Infection of nails and skin, particularly of the groin and feet	Worldwide; anthropophilic
Microsporum audouinii	Infection of scalp and glabrous skin in children; rarely infects adults	Worldwide but primarily in Africa, Rumania, and Haiti; rarely in North America or Europe; anthropophilic
Microsporum canis	Infection of scalp, glabrous skin, and occasionally nails in children	Worldwide; zoophilic (dogs, cats)
Microsporum ferrugineum	Infection of scalp	Africa, east Asia, eastern Europe; anthropophilic
Microsporum gypseum	Infection of scalp and glabrous skin	Worldwide; geophilic
Microsporum persicolor	Infection of scalp, glabrous skin, and feet	Worldwide; zoophilic (small rodents)
Phaeoannellomyces (Exophiala) werneckii	Infection (tinea nigra) of palms of hands and, occasionally, the dorsa of the feet	Tropical areas of Central and South America, Africa, and Asia; southeastern U.S.

(continued)

Microbes of Humans

Microbes of Humans

Table 2.2 Fungal pathogens and geographic distribution *(continued)*

Fungi	Human body sites	Geographic distribution
Piedraia hortae	Infection (black piedra) of scalp hair; less commonly beard, axillary, or pubic hairs	Tropical regions of Africa, Asia, and Central and South America
Trichophyton concentricum	Infection of glabrous skin	Oceania, Southeast Asia, Central and South America; anthropophilic
Trichophyton megninii	Infection of glabrous skin, scalp, and beard	Europe (particularly Portugal and Italy), Africa; rare in Western Hemisphere; anthropophilic
Trichophyton mentagrophytes	Infection of all body surfaces including nails, hair, and (particularly) feet	Worldwide; anthropophilic or zoophilic (primarily small mammals)
Trichophyton rubrum	Infection of skin and nails (most common pathogenic dermatophyte)	Worldwide; anthropophilic
Trichophyton schoenleinii	Infection of scalp (favus) and occasionally nails and skin	Primarily in Eurasia and Africa; anthropophilic
Trichophyton soudanense	Infection of scalp and hair	Central and West Africa; anthropophilic
Trichophyton tonsurans	Infection of scalp (most common pathogen), as well as skin and nails	Worldwide, particularly in the U.S. and Latin America; anthropophilic
Trichophyton verrucosum	Infection of scalp, beard, nails, and other skin surfaces	Worldwide distribution; zoophilic (cattle, horses)

Trichophyton violaceum	Infection of scalp, as well as glabrous skin, nails, and soles of feet	North Africa, Middle East, Europe, South America, and Mexico; anthropophilic
Zygomycosis		
Apophysomyces elegans	Rare cause of traumatic zygomycosis	Worldwide
Absidia corymbifera	Pulmonary infections, as well as infections of the skin, meninges, and kidneys	Worldwide
Basidiobolus ranarum	Subcutaneous zygomycosis of limbs, chest, back, or buttocks	Worldwide
Conidiobolus coronatus	Subcutaneous zygomycosis of nasal mucosa, with spread into adjacent tissues	Worldwide, primarily in tropical and subtropical areas
Cunninghamella bertholletiae	Rare cause of pulmonary or disseminated zygomycosis	Primarily in Mediterranean or subtropical areas
Mucor spp.	Uncommon cause of disseminated zygomycosis	Worldwide
Rhizomucor pusillus	Pulmonary, disseminated, or cutaneous zygomycosis	Worldwide

(continued)

Microbes of Humans

Microbes of Humans

Table 2.2 Fungal pathogens and geographic distribution (*continued*)

Fungi	Human body sites	Geographic distribution
Rhizopus spp.	Primary cause of invasive zygomycosis, particularly involving spread from nasopharynx to brain	Worldwide
Saksenaea vasiformis	Occasional cause of rhinocerebral zygomycosis, as well as involvement of bone, skin, and subcutaneous tissues	Worldwide
Mycetoma		
Acremonium spp. (*A. falciforme, A. kiliense, A. recifei*)	Mycetoma (*A. falciforme* is the second most common cause in U.S.)	India, Thailand, U.S. Africa, Rumania, Venezuela, Brazil
Curvularia spp. (*C. geniculata, C. lunata*)	Mycetoma (*C. geniculata* in dogs)	U.S. (*C. geniculata*); Senegal (*C. lunata*)
Exophiala jeanselmei	Mycetoma; subcutaneous phaeohyphomycosis; peritonitis	U.S. Europe, India, Malaya, Thailand, Argentina
Leptosphaeria spp. (*L. senegalensis, L. tompkinsii*)	Mycetoma	Northern tropical West Africa (especially Senegal and Mauritania), India
Madurella spp. (*M. grisea, M. mycetomatis*)	Mycetoma	Venezuela, Argentina, Paraguay, Chile, Brazil, British West Indies, India, Zaire (*M. grisea*); Venezuela, Argentina, Rumania, India, Sudan, Senegal, Somalia (*M. mycetomatis*)

Neotestudina rosatii	Mycetoma	Australia, Cameroon, Guinea, Senegal, Somalia
Pseudallescheria boydii	Mycetoma (most common cause in U.S.)	U.S., Mexico, Venezuela, Argentina, Uruguay, India, Rumania
Pyrenochaeta romeroi	Mycetoma	Somalia, Senegal, India, South America
Moniliaceous fungi		
Aspergillus spp.	*A. fumigatus*, *A. flavus*, and *A. niger* are the most common pathogens; capable of colonization, invasive disease, toxicoses, or allergy	Worldwide
Fusarium spp.	*F. solani*, *F. oxysporum*, and *F. moniliforme* are the most common pathogens; cause eye infection and, less commonly, systemic infection, sinusitis, skin and nail infection, and mycetoma	Worldwide
Paecilomyces spp.	*P. variotii* and *P. lilacinus* are the most common pathogens; cause keratitis and, less commonly, endocarditis, sinusitis, nephritis, pulmonary infection, and skin and soft tissue infection	Worldwide

(continued)

Microbes of Humans

Table 2.2 Fungal pathogens and geographic distribution *(continued)*

Fungi	Human body sites	Geographic distribution
Penicillium spp.	With the exception of *P. marneffei*, most isolates are contaminants	Worldwide
Scopulariopsis spp.	*S. brevicaulis* is the most common pathogen, as well as a frequent lab contaminant; infection of toenails and (less commonly) fingernails	Worldwide
Dematiaceous fungi		
Alternaria spp.	Phaeohyphomycosis of bone, skin, ears, eyes, sinuses, and urinary tract (this genus and other dematiaceous fungi are frequently isolated as lab contaminants)	Worldwide
Aureobasidium pullulans	Phaeohyphomycosis of nail, skin, subcutaneous, and deep tissues	Worldwide
Bipolaris spp.	*B. australiensis, B. hawaiiensis,* and *B. spicifera* are associated with infection of meninges, eye, sinuses, respiratory tract, and subcutaneous tissues	Worldwide

Chaetomium spp.	Phaeohyphomycosis of skin, nails, and deep tissues	Worldwide
Cladophialophora spp.	Chromoblastomycosis (*C. carrionii* is the most common cause in Africa, Australia, and Madagascar)	Worldwide
Cladosporium spp.	Cutaneous, subcutaneous, and eye infections	Worldwide
Curvularia spp.	Common cause of fungal sinusitis and keratitis; less commonly associated with other infections	Worldwide
Dactylaria spp.	Opportunistic pathogen	Worldwide
Exserohilum spp.	*E. longirostratum, E. mcginnisii, and E. rostratum* are associated with phaeohyphomycosis of skin, subcutaneous tissue, and sinuses	Worldwide
Fonsecaea spp.	*F. compacta* is the most common cause of chromoblastomycosis; *F. pedrosoi* is a rare cause	Worldwide
Lasiodiplodia theobromae	Keratitis; rare cause of subcutaneous infection	Worldwide

(continued)

Microbes of Humans

Microbes of Humans

Table 2.2 Fungal pathogens and geographic distribution *(continued)*

Fungi	Human body sites	Geographic distribution
Lecythophora spp.	*L. hoffmannii* and *L. mutabilis* cause subcutaneous phaeohyphomycosis, endocarditis, and peritonitis	Worldwide
Nattrassia mangiferae	Phaeohyphomycosis of skin and nail	Worldwide
Phialemonium spp.	*P. curvatum* and *P. obovatum* cause infection of subcutaneous tissues, endocarditis, and peritonitis	Worldwide
Phialophora spp.	*P. verrucosa* is the leading cause of chromoblastomycosis in North America; phaeohyphomycosis, endocarditis, keratitis, osteomyelitis, and opportunistic infections	Worldwide
Phoma spp.	Phaeohyphomycosis involving skin and subcutaneous tissues, lung, cornea, and sinuses	Worldwide
Rhinocladiella spp.	*R. aquaspersa* is a rare cause of chromoblastomycosis	Brazil, Mexico
Scytalidium dimidiatum	Nail and skin infections	Worldwide
Wangiella dermatitidis	Phaeohyphomycosis of skin and subcutaneous tissues	Worldwide

Table 2.3 Parasitic pathogens and geographic distribution

Parasites	Human body sites[a]	Geographic distribution
Protozoa: amoebae		
Acanthamoeba spp.	Brain, skin, eye, lungs	Worldwide
Balamuthia mandrillaris	Brain, CSF	Worldwide
Blastocystis hominis	Small and large intestine	Worldwide
Endolimax nana	Lumen of colon and cecum	Worldwide
Entamoeba histolytica	Lumen of colon and cecum; extraintestinal sites include liver, lung, brain, skin	Worldwide
Entamoeba hartmanni	Lumen of colon and cecum	Worldwide
Entamoeba coli	Lumen of colon and cecum	Worldwide
Iodamoeba butschlii	Lumen of colon and cecum	Worldwide
Naegleria fowleri	Brain, CSF	Worldwide
Protozoa: flagellates		
Chilomastix mesnili	Primarily large intestine	Worldwide
Dientamoeba fragilis	Colon	Worldwide

(continued)

Microbes of Humans

Table 2.3 Parasitic pathogens and geographic distribution *(continued)*

Parasites	Human body sites[a]	Geographic distribution
Giardia lamblia	Small intestine	Worldwide
Leishmania chagasi, L. donovani, L. infantium	Visceral leishmaniasis: amastigotes in bone marrow or aspirates from spleen, lymph nodes, or liver	*L. chagasi* in Central and South America; *L. donovani* in China, India, Middle East, Africa; *L. infantum* in North Africa, Southwest Asia, Mediterranean, Europe
Leishmania tropica, L. braziliensis, L. major, other spp.	Cutaneous leishmaniasis: amastigotes in cutaneous lesions	Many species worldwide
Trichomonas hominis	Cecum	Worldwide
Trichomonas tenex	Mouth	Worldwide
Trichomonas vaginalis	Vagina, urethra, prostate	Worldwide
Trypanosoma brucei gambiense	Trypomastigotes in blood, CSF, brain, lymph nodes, and spleen	West Central Africa
Trypanosoma brucei rhodesiense	As with *T. b. gambiense*	East Central Africa
Trypanosoma cruzi	Trypomastigotes in blood; amastigotes and epimastigotes in pseudocysts in cardiac and smooth muscle, glial cells, and phagocytes	Western Hemisphere from southern U.S. south to Argentina

Protozoa: ciliates		
Balantidium coli	Colon	Widespread in tropics
Protozoa: apicomplexans		
Babesia spp.	Parasitize erythrocytes	*B. microti* in North America and Europe; other species (e.g., *B. divergens, B. equi*) with worldwide distribution
Cryptosporidium parvum	Intracellular parasite of intestinal and respiratory epithelial cells; biliary tree	Worldwide
Cyclospora cayetanensis	Intracellular parasite of jejunum enterocytes	North, Central, and South America; Caribbean, Africa, Southeast Asia, Eastern and Western Europe, Australia
Isospora belli	Intracellular parasite of duodenum and jejunum	Worldwide
Plasmodium falciparum	Ring forms and gametocytes infect erythrocytes of all ages; trophozoites and schizonts not typically seen in peripheral blood; no persistent exoerythrocytic stage	Widely distributed in tropics and subtropics, particularly Africa and Asia; chloroquine-resistant strains reported in Africa, Asia, Papua New Guinea, Solomon Islands, Indian subcontinent, and South America

(continued)

Microbes of Humans

Table 2.3 Parasitic pathogens and geographic distribution *(continued)*

Parasites	Human body sites[a]	Geographic distribution
Plasmodium malariae	Trophozoites, schizonts, and gametocytes parasitize mature erythrocytes; no persistent exoerythrocytic stage, but low-level parasitemia can persist for years	Present in tropics and subtropics (e.g., tropical Africa, India, Myanmar, Sri Lanka, Malaysia, Indonesia) but less common than other plasmodia
Plasmodium ovale	Trophozoites, schizonts, and gametocytes parasitize reticulocytes; hypnozoites persist in hepatic parenchymal cells	Present in tropical Africa (particularly in West Africa), New Guinea, Philippines; also reported in Southeast Asia
Plasmodium vivax	Trophozoites, schizonts, and gametocytes in erythrocytes, with preference for reticulocytes; hypnozoites persist in hepatic parenchymal cells	Worldwide; predominant species in temperate areas; less commonly in tropics such as West Africa; chloroquine-resistant strains reported in Indonesia
Sarcocystis spp.	Intracellular parasite of intestinal epithelium; cysts in skeletal and cardiac muscle	Worldwide
Toxoplasma gondii	Cysts in skeletal muscle, myocardium, brain; tachyzoites in blood, CSF, ocular fluid, bronchoalveolar lavage fluid	Worldwide

Protozoa: microsporidia

Encephalitozoon spp.	Parasite of intestinal enterocytes and macrophages of lamina propria; kidney, liver, and bronchial epithelium; uroepithelium; cells of cornea and respiratory tract	Worldwide
Enterocytozoon bieneusi	Primarily in epithelium of the small intestine and biliary tree; also in respiratory epithelium, liver, and pancreas	Worldwide
Nosema spp.	Eye, muscle	Worldwide
Pleistophora spp.	Muscle	Unknown
Trachipleistophora spp.	Eye, muscle, sinuses	Unknown
Vittaforma spp.	Eye	Unknown

Nematodes

Ancylostoma duodenale	Adults: small intestine; eggs: feces	Southern Europe, northern Africa, China, India, Japan
Angiostrongylus cantonensis	Larvae and young adults in CSF	Thailand, Tahiti, Taiwan; less commonly in Cuba, Central America, and Louisiana

(continued)

Microbes of Humans

Microbes of Humans

Table 2.3 Parasitic pathogens and geographic distribution (*continued*)

Parasites	Human body sites[a]	Geographic distribution
Angiostrongylus costricensis	Adults: terminal ileus, cecum, colon, regional lymph nodes, mesenteric arteries; larvae and eggs in surrounding tissue	Costa Rica, Mexico, Central and South America
Anisakis spp.	Larvae: wall of stomach or intestine; occasionally in extraintestinal sites	Worldwide where uncooked fish is consumed
Ascaris lumbricoides	Adults: small intestine; larvae: small intestine, liver, lungs; eggs: feces	Worldwide (particularly in warm, moist regions)
Brugia malayi	Adults: lymphatic system; microfilaria: blood	Southeast Asia, Philippines, Korea, southern China, India
Brugia timori	Adults: lymphatic system; microfilaria: blood	Lesser Sunda Islands of Indonesian archipelago
Capillaria hepatica	Adults: liver	Worldwide
Capillaria philippinensis	Adults: intestine; eggs: feces; larvae: occasionally found in feces	Philippines, Thailand, Japan, Taiwan, Egypt, Iran, Colombia
Dirofilaria immitis	Larvae in pulmonary nodules	Worldwide in tropical, subtropical, and warm temperate regions; southern coastal and southeastern U.S.
Dracunculus medinensis	Adults in cutaneous lesions	Worldwide

Enterobius vermicularis	Adults: cecum, appendix, colon, rectum; eggs: deposited in perianal area	Worldwide
Eustrongylides spp.	Adults: abdominal cavity, intestines	Worldwide where uncooked fish is consumed (rare)
Gnathostoma spp.	Larvae: tissues	China, Philippines, Thailand, Japan
Loa loa	Adults: subcutaneous tissue; microfilaria: blood	Equatorial rain forests of Central and West Africa
Mansonella ozzardi	Adults: subcutaneous tissue; microfilaria: blood	Central America (e.g., Mexico, Panama) and northern part of South America, West Indies
Mansonella perstans	Adults: abdominal cavity, mesenteries, peritoneal tissues; microfilaria: blood	Africa, South America, some Caribbean islands
Mansonella streptocerca	Adults: subcutaneous tissues; microfilaria: skin snips	Rain forests of Central and West Africa (e.g., Zaire, Ghana, Nigeria, Cameroon)
Necator americanus	Adults: small intestine; eggs: feces	Western Hemisphere, Central and South Africa, southern Asia, India, Melanesia, Polynesia
Onchocerca volvulus	Adults: subcutaneous nodules; microfilaria: skin snips; occasionally blood or urine	Africa, Yemen, Central America (Mexico, Guatemala), South America (Venezuela, Colombia, Ecuador, Brazil)

(continued)

Microbes of Humans

Table 2.3 Parasitic pathogens and geographic distribution (*continued*)

Parasites	Human body sites[a]	Geographic distribution
Strongyloides stercoralis	Adults: small intestine; larvae: feces	Worldwide (particularly in warm, moist regions)
Toxocara spp.	Visceral larva migrans; larvae found in various tissues including liver, eye, and central nervous system	Worldwide (particularly in warm, moist regions)
Trichinella spiralis	Adults: intestines; larvae: encyst in muscle tissue	Worldwide (primarily in Europe and North America; less commonly in tropical areas)
Trichostrongylus spp.	Adults: small intestine; eggs: feces	Worldwide (associated with herbivorous animals)
Trichuris trichiura	Adults: large intestine, cecum, appendix; eggs: feces	Worldwide (particularly in warm, moist regions)
Wuchereria bancrofti	Adults: lymphatic system; microfilaria: blood	Widespread in tropics and subtropics
Trematodes		
Clonorchis sinensis	Adults: bile ducts; eggs: feces	China, Taiwan, Japan, Korea, Vietnam

Dicrocoelium dendriticum	Adults: bile ducts; eggs: feces	Europe, former USSR, northern Africa, northern Asia, Far East, Western Hemisphere
Echinostoma hortense	Adults: small intestine; eggs: feces	Southeast Asia
Fasciola hepatica	Adults: bile ducts; eggs: feces	Worldwide (particularly in sheep-raising countries)
Fasciolopsis buski	Adults: small intestine; eggs: feces	China, Taiwan, Thailand, Indonesia, India, Bangladesh, Cambodia, Myanmar, Vietnam
Gastrodiscoides hominis	Adults: cecum, colon; eggs: feces	India, Southeast Asia, former USSR
Heterophyes heterophyes	Adults: small intestine; eggs: feces	Nile River delta, Turkey, East and Southeast Asia
Metagonimus yokogawai	Adults: small intestine; eggs: feces	China, Japan, Southeast Asia, Balkan states
Metorchis conjunctus	Adults: bile ducts; eggs: feces	Canada
Nanophyetus salmincola	Adults: small intestine; eggs: feces	Northwest North America
Neodiplostomum seoulense	Adults: small intestine; eggs: feces	Southeast Asia
Opisthorchis spp.	Adults: bile ducts; eggs: feces	*O. viverrine*: Thailand, Laos; *O. felineus*: Eastern Europe, former USSR

(continued)

Microbes of Humans

Table 2.3 Parasitic pathogens and geographic distribution *(continued)*

Parasites	Human body sites[a]	Geographic distribution
Paragonimus westermani	Adults: lung parenchyma; occasionally in abdominal wall, connective tissues, and organs; subcutaneous tissues; brain; eggs: feces or sputum	China, Japan, Korea; other species in Latin America, Southeast Asia, Africa
Phaneropsolus bonnei	Adults: small intestine; eggs: feces	Southeast Asia
Prosthodendrium molenkampi	Adults: small intestine; eggs: feces	Southeast Asia
Pygidiopsis summa	Adults: small intestine; eggs: feces	Southeast Asia
Schistosoma haematobium	Adults: venous plexuses of bladder and rectum; eggs: biopsy of bladder wall or rectum, feces	Africa, Madagascar, Arabian peninsula, Iraq, Iran, Syria, Lebanon, Turkey, India
Schistosoma japonicum	Adults: venous plexuses of small intestine; eggs: feces, rectal biopsy	China, Philippines, Indonesia, Thailand
Schistosoma mansoni	Adults: venous plexuses of colon and lower ileum; hepatic portal system; eggs: feces, rectal biopsy	Africa, Madagascar, Arabian peninsula, Caribbean islands, South America (Brazil, Suriname, Venezuela)
Schistosoma mekongi	Adults: venous plexuses of small intestine; eggs: feces, rectal biopsy	Laos, Cambodia, Thailand

Cestodes

Diphyllobothrium latum	Adults: small intestine; eggs and proglottids: feces	Fish tapeworm in cold lakes of northern Europe, Baltic countries, North America, Japan; other species found in Alaska, Peru, and Japan
Dipylidium caninum	Adults: small intestine; eggs and proglottids: feces	Worldwide (dog tapeworm)
Echinococcus granulosus	Unilocular hydatid disease; larvae form cysts in any tissue including liver, lung, and brain	Sheep-raising countries (e.g., Australia, New Zealand, southern Africa, southern South America); parts of Europe, North America, and the Orient
Echinococcus multilocularis	Multilocular hydatid disease; larvae form cysts in any tissue, particularly liver	Northern Europe, Japan, China, India, North America (Alaska, Canada, northern midwestern U.S.)
Echinococcus vogeli	Polycystic hydatid disease; larvae form cysts primarily in liver	Latin America
Hymenolepis diminuta	Adults: small intestine; eggs: feces	Worldwide (rat tapeworm)
Hymenolepis nana	Adults: small intestine; eggs: feces	Worldwide (dwarf tapeworm)
Spirometra mansoni	Larvae migrate to brain	China, Japan, Korea, Vietnam
Spirometra mansonoides	Larvae migrate in subcutaneous tissues	U.S.

(continued)

Microbes of Humans

Microbes of Humans

Table 2.3 Parasitic pathogens and geographic distribution (*continued*)

Parasites	Human body sites[a]	Geographic distribution
Taenia multiceps	Larva form cysts in subcutaneous tissues, muscle, eye, and central nervous system	Sheep-raising countries
Taenia saginata	Adults: small intestine; eggs and proglottids: feces	Worldwide (beef tapeworm)
Taenia solium	Adults: small intestine; eggs and proglottids: feces; larvae (*Cysticercus cellulosae*) form cysts in various tissues including brain and muscle	Worldwide (pork tapeworm), particularly in middle European countries, Mexico, Latin America, India, China

[a]CSF, cerebrospinal fluid.

Specimen Collection and Transport

The most important aspects of microbiological testing are collection of the right specimen and transport of the specimen to the testing site in a manner that ensures the reliability of the diagnostic procedure (e.g., culture, microscopy, and antigen or antibody tests). The following guidelines should be useful for most medically important organisms and the most commonly submitted specimens. For special testing situations, selection of the appropriate diagnostic tests requires communication between the microbiologist and physician. For additional information about specific organisms or specimen types, please consult the general references listed in the Bibliography, particularly Miller's *A Guide to Specimen Management in Clinical Microbiology*.

Organism-Specific Guidelines for Specimen Collection and Transport

BACTERIOLOGY
General Guidelines
1. Appropriate safety precautions must be used for the collection, transport, and initial processing of all specimens.

2. Many infections are caused by the patient's indigenous microbial population. For this reason, it is important to avoid contamination of the specimen with these organisms.

3. Specimens should be collected from the areas of actively replicating organisms. Typically, pus contains relatively few viable organisms. A more appropriate specimen would be scrapings or a biopsy specimen from the wall of an abscess.

4. The quantity of specimen collected must be sufficient to ensure that all requested tests (cultures, microscopy, antigen tests, nucleic acid probes, and amplification tests) can be performed properly. If only a limited amount of specimen can be collected, tests should be performed selectively.

5. As a general rule, swabs collect an inadequate quantity of specimen, are easily contaminated, and are subject to drying with subsequent loss of most microbes.

6. Transport of specimens should maintain the viability of the etiologic agent (if culture is performed) and prevent overgrowth with contaminating organisms.

Gram-Positive Cocci

***Enterococcus* spp.** Blood, peritoneal fluid, urine, and wound specimens collected for culture. No special precautions needed for collection or transport. Resistant to desiccation and temperature changes; can be stored at 4°C for prolonged times.

***Peptostreptococcus* spp.** Blood, other normally sterile fluids, and aspirates of abscesses and wound exudates collected for culture. Swab specimens should be discouraged. Transport in appropriate system that maintains a moist, anaerobic atmosphere. Maintain at ambient temperature until the specimen is processed.

***Staphylococcus* spp.** Blood, other normally sterile fluids, urine, abscesses and wound exudates, respiratory and vaginal secretions, and catheters collected for culture. No special precautions are needed for collection or transport. Resistant to desiccation and temperature changes; can be stored at 4°C for prolonged times.

***Streptococcus,* Group A.** Throat swab, blood, other normally sterile fluids, and abscesses and wound exudates collected for culture. Care must be used to sample the involved area in pharyngitis and to avoid contamination with saliva (contains inhibitory bacteria). No special precautions are needed for collection or transport. Resistant to desiccation and temperature changes; can be stored at 4°C for prolonged times. Throat swab can be collected for direct antigen test (other specimens not acceptable). Serum collected for serological tests.

***Streptococcus,* Group B.** Vaginal secretions, rectal swabs, urine, cerebrospinal fluid (CSF), respiratory secretions, blood, and abscesses and wound exudates collected for culture. Specimens should be transported in a moist, non-nutritive environment to prevent overgrowth of other bacteria. Transport on dry swabs preferred for vaginal, rectal, and CSF specimens submitted for direct antigen tests (rapid, specific but insensitive test used to supplement but not replace culture).

Streptococcus pneumoniae. Blood, other normally sterile fluids (particularly CSF), respiratory secretions, and aspirates of sinuses and middle ear collected for culture. Labile organism; avoid desiccation or extremes in temperature (including storage of specimens at 4°C). Organism undergoes autolysis, so specimens should be processed immediately.

***Streptococcus*, Viridans Group.** Blood and aspirates of abscesses and wound exudates collected for culture. Specimens should be transported in blood culture bottles or a moist, nonnutritive environment.

Gram-Positive Bacilli

***Actinomyces* spp.** Aspirates of periodontal abscesses and sinus tracts in the face, neck, thorax, abdomen, and vagina are collected for culture. Granular colonies ("sulfur granules"), if present, should be collected. Avoid contamination of the specimen with organisms (including *Actinomyces* spp.) colonizing adjacent mucosal surfaces. Transport in an appropriate system that maintains a moist, anaerobic atmosphere. Maintain at ambient temperature until the specimen is processed. Granules should be crushed for culture and microscopy.

Arcanobacterium haemolyticum. Specimens for culture include throat swabs and aspirates from skin ulcers. No special precautions are needed for collection or transport.

Bacillus anthracis. Observe appropriate safety precautions for collection and transport of all specimens. Swab vesicular exudate in early cutaneous lesions or collect fluid under the edge of eschar if present; collect blood for intestinal or pulmonary anthrax, as well as feces and respiratory secretions, respectively. All specimens should be directly transported to the lab by the individual responsible for collection. Organism is resistant to desiccation and temperature extremes. Direct detection by PCR is a research tool; serological testing is used only to monitor response to vaccination.

Bacillus cereus. Specimens submitted for culture include food but not stool (food poisoning), exudate from eye (traumatic or surgical ocular infections), and blood (systemic infections). No special precautions are needed for collection or transport; organism resistant to desiccation and temperature extremes.

Clostridium botulinum. Submit stool and the implicated food for culture; food and the patient's stool and serum are tested for toxin activity. Wound botulism is confirmed by wound culture or detection of toxin activity in wound exudate or serum. Specimens for culture are transported in an appropriate system that maintains a moist, anaerobic atmosphere. Maintain at ambient temperature until the specimen is processed.

Clostridium difficile. Submit stool for toxin testing (active disease) or culture (asymptomatic colonization or active disease). Specimens transported as for *C. botulinum*. Specimens for toxin assay can be stored at 4°C for 3 days or at −70°C for longer periods; do not store at −20°C.

Clostridium perfringens. Specimens submitted for culture include blood, exudates, tissue specimens, and food implicated in food poisoning (not feces). Specimens transported as for *C. botulinum*.

Clostridium tetani. Wound specimens can be cultured, but typically this organism is not isolated. Lab tests are used primarily to exclude other similar diseases.

Corynebacterium diphtheriae. Specimens include nasopharyngeal swab, or swab or aspirate from under membrane covering ulcerative lesions; collection of multiple specimens is optimum. Bacteria are relatively resistant to desiccation and temperature changes. Can be transported with no special precautions or on Amies semisolid medium. If culture is delayed more than 24 h, silica gel transport medium recommended.

Corynebacterium jeikeium. Blood is collected for culture. Avoid contamination with members of the skin flora (common source of this organism). Inoculate specimen directly into blood culture bottles.

Corynebacterium urealyticum. Should be suspected in patients with alkaline urine and stone formation. Urine or urinary calculi are collected for culture. Transport specimen rapidly to laboratory or store at 4°C to prevent overgrowth of contaminants.

***Corynebacterium*, Other spp.** Blood, CSF, prosthetic devices, and catheter specimens are collected for culture. Care must be used to avoid contamination with members of skin flora. No special precautions are needed for specimen transport.

Erysipelothrix rhusiopathiae. Perform full-thickness biopsy at leading edge of skin lesion; superficial samples collected from the lesion or skin surface are of no value; blood is collected if there is evidence of systemic disease (e.g., endocarditis). No special precautions are needed for specimen transport.

Listeria monocytogenes. CSF, blood, amniotic fluid, placenta, or fetal tissue is collected for culture. CSF and tissue can also be processed for PCR tests (research tool). Specimens can be transported or stored at 4°C; listeriae survive and grow at this temperature.

***Propionibacterium* spp.** Blood, CSF, prosthetic devices, and catheter specimens are collected for culture. Avoid contamination with members of the skin flora. Transport in an appropriate system that maintains a moist, anaerobic atmosphere and prevents overgrowth of contaminants. Maintain at ambient temperature until the specimen is processed.

Acid-Fast Bacilli

Mycobacterium tuberculosis. Observe appropriate safety precautions for collection and transport of all specimens. Respiratory specimens, gastric lavage fluid (pediatric patients), pleural fluid, CSF, urine, tissues (minimum, 1 g), and blood are collected for culture. Collect 5 to 10 ml of respiratory or lavage specimens on three consecutive days. Neutralize lavage fluid with sodium carbonate before transport to the lab. At least 2 to 5 ml of CSF must be collected; 30 to 40 ml of first-voided urine is collected on three to five consecutive days. Collect blood in Isolator system or Bactec 13A bottle. No 24-h pooled specimens (respiratory, urine) are acceptable. If specimen transport exceeds 1 h, store specimen at 4°C to prevent overgrowth of contaminants. Respiratory specimens are collected for DNA amplification and hybridization. Immunodiagnostic tests for antigen or antibody are available but of limited utility.

Mycobacterium leprae. Culture is not performed; acid-fast organisms are commonly seen in biopsied skin lesions from patients with lepromatous leprosy but not with tuberculoid leprosy. Highest yields are in biopsy specimens from rim of lesion. Skin test is diagnostic in patients with tuberculoid form but not useful in lepromatous form.

***Mycobacterium*, Other spp.** Respiratory specimens, pleural fluid, CSF, urine, tissues, blood, wound exudates, and feces are collected for culture. Samples from wounds and skin ulcers should be transported in Amies or Stuart's medium; dry specimens are unacceptable. Culture of feces is controversial and should be done only for *M. avium* complex. Fecal specimens must be refrigerated until processed. All other specimens should be collected and transported as for *M. tuberculosis*. Direct detection tests currently not used.

***Nocardia* spp.** Respiratory specimens, CSF, cutaneous lesions, and wound exudates are collected for culture (blood cultures are rarely positive). Specimens should be rapidly transported to the lab for processing because *Nocardia* spp. cannot tolerate refrigeration.

Rhodococcus equi. Respiratory specimens and aspirates for abscesses and wounds are submitted for culture. No special precautions are needed for specimen collection or transport.

Gram-Negative Cocci and Coccobacilli

Moraxella catarrhalis. Respiratory specimens, tympanocentesis fluid, and sinus aspirates are collected for culture. Specimens should be processed immediately, although data on survival of organism is not available.

Neisseria gonorrhoeae. Specimens for culture include eye exudate, pharyngeal swab, urethral specimens collected at least 1 h after urination, vaginal secretions, rectal swabs (avoid gross fecal contamination), synovial fluid, blood, and skin lesions. Specimens should be inoculated directly onto selective media or rapidly transported to lab in Stuart's or Amies medium. Survival on transport medium beyond 6 h is poor. Avoid exposure to temperature extremes including refrigeration at 4°C. Exposure of blood specimens to sodium polyanetholsulfonate (SPS) should be avoided or minimized (use SPS-free culture media, add gelatin to the medium, or process in the lysis-centrifugation system). Samples for direct DNA amplification and probe testing include genital specimens and first-voided urine. Specimens must be collected and transported in the system recommended by the individual manufacturers.

Neisseria meningitidis. Specimens for culture include CSF, blood, respiratory specimens, and skin lesions. Nasopharyngeal swabs are better than oropharyngeal swabs for detection of carriers. Observe the same precautions for specimen collection and transport as with *N. gonorrhoeae*.

DNA amplification tests are not commercially available. Antigen tests are available for CSF specimens but are not commonly used (poor sensitivity).

Gram-Negative Bacilli

***Aeromonas* spp.**   Blood, wound specimens, and feces are collected for culture. No special precautions are needed for collection or transport; bacteria can survive up to 5 days in glycerol-buffered saline. Cary-Blair or other transport media can be used for fecal specimens. Rectal swabs should not be processed.

***Bacteroides* spp.**   Specimens submitted for culture include aspirates from abscesses in the brain, respiratory tract, abdominal cavity, pelvic space, and wounds, as well as blood. Specimen collection on swabs should be discouraged. Transport in an appropriate system that maintains a moist, anaerobic atmosphere; maintain at ambient temperature until the specimen is processed. Do not refrigerate.

Bordetella pertussis.   Nasopharyngeal (NP) aspirates are collected for culture; superior to NP swabs and throat swabs; "cough" plates should not be collected. If swabs are used, calcium alginate is superior, Dacron fiber swabs are slightly less good, and cotton swabs are toxic for the organism. Dacron fiber swabs must be used for specimens collected for PCR testing (alginate and aluminum shafts are inhibitory). Specimens should be cultured at the time of collection. If this is not feasible, transport in special medium (Regan-Lowe), Casamino Acids broth if <2 h, or Amies medium with charcoal if 2 to 24 h. Use Regan-Lowe medium for shipping to distant labs. Transport at ambient temperature; culture yield is lower at 4°C.

***Brucella* spp.**   Specimens include blood, bone marrow, spleen and liver biopsy specimens, abscesses, and infected tissues. Maintain in a moist environment; refrigerate at 4°C if the specimen cannot be immediately processed. Blood is collected for antibody testing.

Burkholderia cepacia.   Specimens include respiratory secretions, blood, peritoneal fluid, synovial fluid, and urine. Hardy organism, so no special transport requirements are needed except that the specimen must be kept moist.

Burkholderia pseudomallei.   Source of nosocomial infections, so care must be used handling specimens and cultures. Specimens include blood and aspirates of abscesses from the lungs, liver, spleen, lymph nodes, skin and soft tissue, and bones. Hardy like *B. cepacia.*

Escherichia coli* and Other Members of the *Enterobacteriaceae. Various specimens collected for culture including blood, other normally sterile fluids, respiratory secretions, urine, feces, and infected tissues. Hardy organism, so no special transport requirements are needed except that the specimen must be kept moist.

Francisella tularensis. Source of nosocomial and laboratory infections, so care must be used in handling specimens and cultures. Specimens include blood and aspirates of ulcers and involved lymph nodes. Ticks or specimens from infected animals can be cultured, but this is rarely done. Specimens must be kept moist; they can be refrigerated but should not be frozen. Blood is collected for antibody testing.

Haemophilus ducreyi. Aspirate of bubo or swab from base of ulcer is collected for culture (microscopy most useful). Specimen must be kept moist and should be processed as quickly as possible. Blood can be collected for antibody detection (specific but insensitive).

Haemophilus influenzae. Blood, sinus aspirates, tympanocentesis fluid, respiratory secretions, and CSF are collected for culture. Avoid contamination with normally colonized body sites. Specimens can be transported in Stuart's medium. Antigen tests for *H. influenzae* type b available but not commonly used now (nonreactive with other serotypes). Serological testing used to monitor response to type b vaccine but not for diagnostic purposes.

***Legionella* spp.** Respiratory specimens and blood are collected for culture. The organism can remain viable for several days at room temperature, although survival decreases in saline. Urine is collected for the antigen test. DNA amplification tests are available for environmental samples (only currently approved use) and patient samples (research labs). Blood is collected for antibody testing. At least 1 liter of water should be collected for environmental samples and mixed with 0.5 ml of 0.1 N sodium thiosulfate. Specimens from faucets and showerheads can be collected with a moist swab and transferred to 3 to 5 ml of water from the receptacle.

Plesiomonas shigelloides. Feces, blood, and CSF are collected for culture. No special precautions are needed for collection or transport; Cary-Blair or other transport media can be used for fecal specimens. Rectal swabs should not be processed.

Porphyromonas **spp.** Specimen collection and transport same as with *Bacteroides* spp.

Prevotella **spp.** Specimen collection and transport same as with *Bacteroides* spp.

Pseudomonas aeruginosa. Specimens include blood, eye, ear, respiratory secretions, urine, and wounds. Hardy organism requiring only that specimens be kept moist. Eye specimens should be inoculated onto appropriate media at time of collection (other more fastidious organisms may be involved).

Salmonella typhi. Blood (and if necessary bone marrow) should be collected in the first week of illness, and stool (possibly urine) specimens should be collected in the second week. Colonization of gallbladder found in long-term carriers. Rectal swabs can be used to screen for carriers. Specimens should be processed rapidly or stored in fecal transport medium.

Salmonella, **Other spp.** Specimens for culture include feces and, less commonly, blood, urine, and infected tissues. Swab specimens should be avoided. Unless processing can be performed within 2 h, specimens should be stored at 4°C or transferred to a fecal transport system and held at ambient temperature.

Shigella **spp.** Specimens for culture include feces and, less commonly, blood. Swab specimens should be avoided. Organism is susceptible to acids, so use of buffered transport system is preferred.

Streptobacillus moniliformis. Blood and joint fluid are collected for culture (very difficult) and microscopic examination; mix with equal volume of 2.5% sodium citrate; avoid inoculation of blood into media with SPS. Antigen tests and serological tests are not currently available.

Vibrio cholerae. Feces or vomitus is collected for culture; transport in Cary-Blair medium at ambient temperature; rectal swabs can be collected but must be kept moist. Buffered glycerol saline or alkaline-peptone water can be used if the specimen is processed within a few hours.

Vibrio parahaemolyticus. Feces, vomitus, or the implicated food may be collected for culture. Specimen transport is the same as with *V. cholerae*.

Vibrio vulnificus. Blood and wound specimens are collected for culture; aspirates or swabs of wounds must be kept moist. No other special precautions needed for collection or transport.

Yersinia enterocolitica. Stool and blood specimens are collected for culture; stool must be kept moist and should be processed within 2 h or transferred to a fecal transport system.

Yersinia pestis. Care must be used in the collection and processing of these specimens. Blood, aspirates from bubo, and wound specimens are collected for culture. Specimens must be kept moist, but no other special precautions are required for collection or transport. Blood is collected for antibody testing.

Curved and Spiral-Shaped Bacilli

Borrelia burgdorferi. Skin biopsy specimen collected just outside the edge of the erythema migrans lesion can be cultured; the organism is rarely isolated from blood or CSF. Organisms not observed in fluids but can be seen in tissue. PCR tests are under development and appear to be the most sensitive. Clinical disease is confirmed by serological testing.

***Borrelia,* Other spp.** Organisms can be observed by light or dark-field microscopy in blood (during febrile episodes); can also be isolated in culture. Serological testing is less helpful (many false-negative reactions).

Campylobacter fetus. Blood (most commonly) is submitted for culture.

***Campylobacter,* Other spp.** Feces is collected for culture. Avoid use of swabs. Transport in Cary-Blair medium and store at 4°C unless processing is immediate. Direct detection by PCR is a research tool; serological testing is used in epidemiological surveys.

Helicobacter pylori. Multiple gastric biopsy specimens from the gastric antrum should be collected. Cimetidine and benzocaine inhibit growth of *H. pylori* and should be avoided; lidocaine is acceptable. Direct detection of urease is generally rapid. The organism rapidly becomes nonviable, particularly if dry, so specimens should be transported in Stuart's transport medium or a variety of media with glycerol or serum; specimens for prolonged transport should be inoculated onto chocolate agar. Viability at 4°C is not maintained beyond 1 week; the specimen can be frozen. Biopsy specimens can be submitted for histological examination or DNA amplification/probe tests (research tools). Noninvasive urease breath test and serological testing are also used.

***Leptospira* spp.** Blood and CSF are collected for culture in tubes with heparin or sodium oxalate (citrate toxic) during the first 10 days of symptoms. Specimens can be stored at 4 to 20°C for up to 1 week before processing. Urine is the specimen of choice after the first week; neutralize if acidic; process immediately or dilute 1:10 with 1% bovine serum albumin (BSA) and store at 4 to 20°C. Direct detection by direct fluorescent antibody (DFA) test or PCR (avoid heparin). Serological testing is also available.

Treponema pallidum. Culture is not performed. Serous fluid (avoid contamination with blood or tissue debris) is collected from primary chancre or aspirated from lesions in the secondary stage for dark-field microscopy or DFA test. PCR is available in research labs. Serological testing (nontreponemal and treponemal) is the procedure of choice for diagnosis.

Mycoplasmas and Obligate Intracellular Bacteria

***Bartonella* spp.** Blood is cultured for patients with disseminated infections; avoid exposure to SPS (use Isolator, neutralize SPS with gelatin, or process in broths with resins). Microscopy is positive only early in infection. PCR is sensitive (research labs). Serological testing is the procedure of choice.

Chlamydia pneumoniae. Throat swabs are collected for culture (difficult to grow compared with other chlamydia). The organism is probably stable, but this is not well defined. The sensitivity and specificity of direct detection tests, DNA-based diagnostic tests, and serological testing are not well defined. Currently, culture and serological testing are recommended.

Chlamydia psittaci. Sputum and blood specimens are collected for culture. The organism is very stable (capable of surviving for months at ambient temperature). Care must be used because this organism is associated with lab-acquired infections. Serological testing is useful.

Chlamydia trachomatis. Specimens submitted for culture include cells lining the cervix or urethra (not exudate), rectal swabs, conjunctiva, nasopharyngeal aspirate, or tracheo-bronchial aspirate (determined by site of infection); first-voided urine (not midstream) can be submitted for DNA testing but is not recommended for culture. The organism is relatively stable, but drying must be avoided. Transport the specimen in 2SP medium (or system recommended by the manufacturer) and store at 4°C if the specimen cannot be processed promptly for culture. Direct detection is by microscopy or immunoassay (both less sensitive than culture). DNA probe and nucleic acid amplification is more sensitive than culture (commercially available; limited indications).

Coxiella burnetti. Extremely stable (survives for months at ambient temperatures), so special transport conditions not required. Culture (in cell cultures) and microscopy (e.g., DFA) are not commonly performed. Blood collected in EDTA or citrate (not heparin) can be used for PCR; sensitive but performed only in research labs. Serological testing is the diagnostic procedure of choice.

***Ehrlichia* spp.** Blood and CSF are collected in EDTA (not heparin). Diagnosis is by PCR (genus- and species-specific tests; sensitive; research labs currently), microscopy (observation of morulae), culture (very insensitive), or serological testing (currently the diagnostic procedure of choice). Microscopy requires immediate preparation of smears before the blood cells deteriorate.

Mycoplasma pneumoniae. Labile organism due to absence of cell wall; extremely sensitive to drying and temperature extremes. Lower respiratory tract specimens must be processed promptly; other specimens are collected with swabs (calcium alginate or Dacron but not cotton) and transported in 2SP or Stuart's medium. Throat swabs are as reliable as expectorated sputum. Specimens can be stored at 4°C for 3 days or frozen at −70°C for prolonged periods. Use dry ice if the specimen is shipped to a reference lab. Culture is slow and insensitive; direct antigen tests are insensitive and nonspecific; DNA probes are insensitive; PCR tests are sensitive but are currently only a research tool. Serological testing is specific but insensitive.

***Rickettsia* spp.** Culture is rarely performed except in reference labs. Blood is collected early in febrile illness for PCR or immunofluorescence; collect in EDTA tubes and store at 4°C until processed. Tissue biopsy specimens for antigen detection (DFA) can also be collected and transported at 4°C. Diagnosis is typically confirmed by serological testing.

VIROLOGY

General Guidelines

1. Transport specimens collected on swabs in a moist environment, such as viral transport medium (e.g., viral Culturette system), 2SP, or other suitable liquid medium. Dried specimens are unacceptable because many viruses, particularly enveloped viruses, will not survive drying.

2. Avoid calcium alginate fiber swabs, charcoal-impregnated swabs, and swabs with wooden shafts, because viral infectivity may be inactivated or toxicity to cell lines may occur.

3. Specimens collected by washings (e.g., nasopharyngeal specimens) may be supplemented with gelatin or BSA to stabilize the viruses.

4. Collect vesicle fluids and skin scrapings without using skin disinfectants, because disinfectants may contaminate the specimen and inactivate the viruses.

5. The base of the vesicle should be swabbed vigorously or scraped to collect cellular material. This generally has a much higher yield than vesicle fluid.

6. Collect blood specimens with citrate or heparin as an anticoagulant. If the specimen is to be processed for PCR tests, avoid heparin because it will bind DNA and cause false-negative reactions.

7. Store specimens for viral culture either at 4 to 8°C or frozen at −70°C. Do not store specimens at −20°C. Specimens should be diluted with an equal volume of 2SP before freezing to protect labile viruses; however, use of other cryopreservatives such as sorbitol or glycerin is not recom-

mended. Ideally, avoid using diluents and freezing, because they reduce the number of infectious viruses inoculated onto cell cultures.

8. Many viruses (e.g., arenaviruses, hantaviruses, filoviruses, lentiviruses, and lyssaviruses) are extremely dangerous. Exercise appropriate care when handling these and other infectious viruses.

Nonenveloped RNA Viruses

Calicivirus (Calicivirus, Norwalk Virus). Feces should be collected; rectal swabs are inadequate specimens. Viral shedding is maximal in the first 2 days of disease; virus is usually not detected after 1 week. Viruses are relatively stable and persist at 4°C for 1 week or more. Culture is sensitive but very slow (not usually performed). Direct detection by electron microscopy (do not use frozen specimens), enzyme immunoassays (the most commonly used test), dot blot hybridization, or RT-PCR (most sensitive test; available in research labs). Serological testing is of limited value.

Enterovirus (Coxsackievirus, Echovirus, Enterovirus, Poliovirus). Viruses stable under a wide range of conditions for long periods (e.g., weeks at 4°C). Rectal and throat swabs, nasal washings, CSF, blood, and urine can be submitted for culture (test of choice for most members of this group); viral transport medium can be used but is not necessary. Direct detection by immunoassays not sensitive; RT-PCR is a promising diagnostic test. Serological testing is of limited value.

Hepatitis A Virus. Fecal samples can be tested if collected during the 2 weeks before symptoms to several days after onset. Feces should be mixed with an equal volume of phosphate-buffered saline and stored at 4°C for up to 16 weeks. Prolonged storage of virus should be at −70°C. Culture is rarely performed. Direct detection by immunoassays is usually difficult unless performed early in disease. Serological testing is the procedure of choice.

Rhinovirus. Virus relatively stable except at acidic pH. Isolated for 1 day before to 6 days after onset of symptoms, with highest level for first 2 days of symptoms. Nasal secretions preferred over throat swabs. Specimens should be transported in viral transport medium; stable at 4°C for at least 1 day; long-term storage at $-70°C$. RT-PCR and sero-logical testing performed primarily in research labs.

Rotavirus. Stool specimens collected during early acute disease (first 3 to 5 days). Viral transport medium or tissue culture medium should not be used (serum components may react with viruses). Specimens should be transported at $4°C$ and not frozen. Culture not typically performed. Direct detection by electron microscopy, enzyme immuno-assays (most commonly performed), or RT-PCR (research lab test). Serological testing available but not commonly performed.

Enveloped RNA Viruses

Arbovirus (California Encephalitis Virus, Dengue Virus, Eastern Equine Encephalitis Virus, Hantavirus, La Crosse Virus, St. Louis Encephalitis Virus, Venezuelan Encephalitis Virus, Western Equine Encephalitis Virus, Yellow Fever Virus). Many viruses fall within this general classification of arthropod-borne or zoonotic infections. Although virus isolation from blood and some tissues can be performed for some infections during the acute phase of disease (e.g., dengue, yellow fever), diagnosis is typically by serological testing.

Arenavirus (Lymphocytic Choriomeningitis Virus, Lassa Fever Virus). Specimens must be handled with great care. Viral isolation must be performed in laboratories with BL-4 facilities. Lymphocytic choriomeningitis (LCM) virus isolated from acute phase sera obtained in first week of illness and CSF if meningeal disease is present. Lassa fever virus isolated from sera and throat washings obtained in first few weeks of illness, as well as spleen, lymph nodes, liver, and kidney tissues obtained at autopsy. Specimens should be stored at $-70°C$ or shipped on dry ice. Serum specimens for antigen or antibody tests should be maintained at $-20°C$ or colder.

Filovirus (Ebola Virus, Marburg Virus). Specimens must be handled as with arenaviruses. Virus recovered from a variety of specimens including sera, throat washings, urine, and involved tissues.

Hepatitis C Virus. Culture not routinely performed; diagnosis made by detecting viral antigens or serological response. Serum should be refrigerated or frozen within 4 to 6 h of collection and maintained at this temperature until tested.

Human Immunodeficiency Virus. Laboratory tests used to assess if patient is infected and level of viral replication. Infection determined by viral culture (rarely necessary), detection of viral nucleic acid or antigens, or serological response. Level of viral replication determined by quantitative RT-PCR or other amplification method.

Influenza Virus. Specimens include nasopharyngeal aspirates (best) or swabs and throat swabs. Collect specimens within 3 days of disease onset. Transport in cell culture medium or nutrient broth supplemented with BSA or gelatin. Specimens should be processed immediately but can be stored at 4°C for up to 4 days; for long-term storage, freeze at −70°C (not −20°C). Direct detection by immunofluorescence, enzyme immunoassay, or electron microscopy (all less sensitive than culture). RT-PCR available (sensitivity same as culture). Serological testing available as confirmatory test.

Measles Virus. Virus is detected a few days before the onset of rash and persists into convalescence. Isolated initially from nasopharyngeal and conjunctival specimens and later from stool, urine, and occasionally CSF. Virus is labile, so transport as for influenza virus. Direct detection by immunofluorescence and enzyme immunoassay. Antigen tests superior to culture. Serological testing available (test of choice).

Mumps Virus. Specimens include saliva (from 9 days before to 8 days after onset of symptoms), urine (for weeks after onset), CSF (in meningitis), and area around Stensen's duct. Virus is unstable, with significant loss within 4 h of specimen collection; it must be stabilized in transport medium with BSA or gelatin. Direct detection by immunofluorescence, enzyme immunoassay, or RT-PCR. Serological testing available.

Paramyxovirus. Specimens include nasopharyngeal aspirates or swabs and throat swabs. Virus excreted primarily in first 2 to 3 days. Transport specimens as for influenza virus. Direct detection by immunofluorescence (test of choice: equivalent to culture), enzyme immunoassays, probe tests, and PCR. Serological testing available as a confirmatory test.

Rabies Virus. Specimens must be handled with great care. Culture not routinely performed. Brain tissue from infected animal submitted for microscopic examination (immunofluorescence; histopathological testing). Human specimens include saliva, cutaneous nerves, or tissue (including medulla, cerebellum, and hippocampus obtained at autopsy). RT-PCR available but rarely needed. Serological testing available.

Respiratory Syncytial Virus. Specimens include nasal aspirates or washings (superior to swabs); virus is unstable, so specimen should be transported in physiologic salt solution with protein stabilizer (BSA or gelatin). Rapid viral loss at elevated temperatures or with freezing. Direct detection by immunofluorescence (superior to culture), enzyme immunoassays, and PCR (reference lab test). Serological testing available.

Rubella Virus. Virus can be cultured, but not typically done. Virus is unstable, as are others in this group. Serological testing is procedure of choice for diagnosing infection or demonstrating immunity.

Nonenveloped DNA Viruses

Adenovirus. Specimens include nasopharyngeal aspirates or swabs, eye exudates, stool or rectal swabs, urine, urethral or cervical swabs, and tissue biopsy specimens. Specimens should be collected early in course of disease. Virus is very stable, so special transport systems not required. Enteric adenoviruses (types 40 and 41) are not cultured. Direct detection by microscopy (immunofluorescence), electron microscopy, enzyme immunoassay, and PCR (available in research labs). Serological testing available.

Erythrovirus (Parvovirus B19). Specimens include blood, nasal or throat washings, cord blood, and amniotic fluid. Virus is very stable (resistant to solvents, detergents, and temperature extremes). Culture is not performed. Direct detection by electron microscopy, dot blot hybridization, and PCR (test of choice). Virus detected in blood 6 days after infection with peak viremia within 2 to 3 days; virus persists for at least 1 week and for up to several months. Serological testing available.

Papillomavirus. Culture and serological testing not performed. Tissue or exfoliated epithelial specimens should be collected for direct hybridization or PCR amplification.

Polyomavirus (JC Virus, BK Virus). Culture and serological testing not routinely performed. Urine, blood, and CSF collected for direct detection by in situ hybridization or PCR (test of choice).

Enveloped DNA Viruses

Cytomegalovirus. Peripheral blood leukocytes, urine, throat washings, and saliva are the most common specimens. Although virus is stable for up to 48 h at 4°C, specimens must be kept moist and should be transported rapidly to the lab; infectivity is lost at −20°C; virus can be frozen in 2SP at −70°C. Direct detection by immunofluorescence or histopathological stains (less sensitive than culture); in situ hybridization, probe tests, and PCR available (rapid, sensitive); serological testing available.

Epstein-Barr Virus. Culture performed with throat gargle (serum-free medium or Hanks balanced salt solution) or citrated blood. Virus is labile, so process immediately or store at −4°C. Direct detection by microscopy (immunofluorescence), in situ hybridization, dot blot hybridization, or PCR (most sensitive test). Serological testing available (initial test of choice).

Hepatitis B Virus. Culture is not performed. Direct detection is possible by microscopy (immunofluorescence), in situ hybridization, and electron microscopy but is rarely performed. PCR test available in research labs. Serum collected for antigen and antibody testing; can be stored at 4°C for 5 days or frozen for longer periods.

Herpes Simplex Virus. Vesicular lesions, blood, and tissues submitted for culture; recovery best in fresh vesicular lesions and lowest at crusted stage. Virus is labile, so process immediately or store at 4°C for up to 48 h. Direct detection by microscopy (immunofluorescence or histopathological stains), in situ hybridization, or PCR (most sensitive test). Serological testing available.

Human Herpesvirus 6. Peripheral blood leukocytes submitted for culture; virus is very labile, so do not freeze. Direct detection by in situ hybridization or PCR; PCR testing with blood, CSF, or saliva. Serological testing available.

Molluscum Contagiosum Virus.   Culture is not available; clinical diagnosis can be confirmed by examining papule microscopically (intracytoplasmic inclusions seen with Giemsa stain).

Varicella-Zoster Virus.   Vesicular lesions, skin scrapings, and tissues submitted for culture; vesicular fluid can be cultured but cannot be used for microscopy; do not culture lesions more than 4 days old or crusted (can be used for antigen tests). Cell-associated virus, so affected area such as base of vesicle must be swabbed aggressively. Virus is labile so must be kept moist and transported rapidly to lab or stored at 4°C. Direct antigen tests by in situ hybridization, microscopy (immunofluorescence), or PCR (most sensitive test). Serological testing available.

MYCOLOGY

General Guidelines

1. Although the recovery of some fungi in clinical specimens is always considered significant (e.g., dermatophytes, dimorphic fungi, *Cryptococcus neoformans*), most fungi are part of the patient's normal flora (e.g., *Candida* spp.) or found in the environment (e.g., most dematiaceous and moniliaceous fungi). Specimens must be carefully collected to avoid contamination with indigenous or exogenous fungi.

2. Bacteria can rapidly overgrow fungi, so care must be used in cleaning the site where the specimen will be collected (e.g., skin surface, nail beds). Transport conditions must be selected to minimize the risk of bacterial overgrowth.

3. Microscopic examination of specimens is important for the rapid detection of a fungal infection and for assessing the significance of an isolate.

Dematiaceous Fungi

Specimens submitted for microscopy and culture include aspirates, scrapings, and tissues. Swabs should not be used because an inadequate quantity of material is recovered and desiccation occurs. Transport medium is unnecessary if the specimen is processed immediately. Serological testing

not available except for *Sporothrix* spp. (discussed below
with dimorphic fungi).

Dermatophytes (*Epidermophyton, Microsporum,* and *Trichophyton* spp.)

Collect infected hairs with sterile forceps (guided by the
use of a Wood's lamp if the suspected dermatophyte is
fluorescent). Endothrix fungi may require the use of a sterile scalpel to collect the hair root. Sample skin lesions at the
active border of the lesion with a sterile scalpel to collect
the sample. Disinfect nails with alcohol before collecting
the sample by clipping or scraping. Do not place hair, skin,
or nail samples in closed tubes. The high humidity fosters
overgrowth of contaminating bacteria.

Dimorphic Fungi (*Blastomyces, Coccidioides, Histoplasma, Paracoccidioides,* and *Sporothrix* spp.)

Process specimens (e.g., respiratory specimens and wound
aspirates) promptly to avoid overgrowth of contaminating
bacteria. Do not use swabs, because these organisms are
susceptible to desiccation. *Histoplasma capsulatum* can be
recovered in blood cultures, particularly from patients with
AIDS and other immunosuppressive diseases. Collect
blood specimens by the lysis-centrifugation system.

Eumycotic Mycetoma Agents

Examine pus, exudate, or biopsy material for the presence
of granules (sclerotia) consisting of the eumycotic agents
and matrix material. Wash the granules with saline containing antibiotics (e.g., penicillin and streptomycin), and then
culture them. Organisms can be visualized by examining
crushed granules microscopically.

Moniliaceous Fungi

Process specimens (e.g., biopsy specimens, lower respiratory secretions, nails, eye specimens) promptly to avoid
overgrowth of contaminating bacteria. Do not transport
specimens on swabs, because organisms are susceptible to
desiccation. Specimens should be examined microscopically and cultured. *Pseudallescheria boydii* and *Fusarium*
spp. are among the few filamentous fungi that can be recovered in blood cultures. Collect blood specimens for these
fungi by the lysis-centrifugation system. Serological tests
are available for some of these fungi.

Pneumocystis carinii

Respiratory specimens should be limited to induced sputa or bronchoscopy specimens. Patients can only rarely expectorate sputum, and throat washings are insensitive. Collect first morning specimens when possible. A 24-h collection is unacceptable. The presence of oral contamination, signified by squamous epithelial cells, does not invalidate the specimen.

Yeast

Yeasts are relatively easy to isolate from clinical specimens, although overgrowth of contaminating bacteria should be avoided. Yeasts are isolated commonly from blood specimens. The lysis-centrifugation system and biphasic culture systems are the most reliable methods of isolating yeasts from blood specimens, although the automated continuous-monitoring systems are reliable for most common yeasts (less reliable for *Candida glabrata* and *Cryptococcus neoformans*). Direct detection includes microscopy (Gram stain, KOH, India ink, calcofluor white) and antigen tests. Serological testing is available for antibodies to *Candida* spp. but is not commonly used.

PARASITOLOGY

General Guidelines

1. Mineral oil and barium bismuth can make examination of fecal specimens impossible, because protozoa and eggs are obscured by these preparations. Collect specimens before treatment, or parasitic examination will have to be delayed for 1 week or more.

2. Antibiotics and antimalarial agents can interfere with examination of fecal specimens for protozoa by reducing the number of parasites for up to 2 weeks.

3. Trophozoites die rapidly in collected stool specimens. If detection of motility is attempted, the specimen must be examined within 30 to 60 min of collection. If this cannot be done, then use of preservatives is recommended.

4. Because most parasitic infections are acquired in the community, specimens should not be processed routinely from patients who have been hospitalized for more than 3 days.

5. A single stool specimen should be collected on three or more consecutive days to detect parasitic infections.

Free-Living Amebae

The laboratory diagnosis of infections due to free-living amebae can be accomplished by isolation of the organisms in culture, microscopy, or serological testing (used primarily to confirm infection and not to make a diagnosis or to guide therapy). Specimens for isolation include CSF, corneal biopsy specimens and scrapings, and brain or other tissues. Collect specimens aseptically and maintain them at room temperature until processed. Specimens can be stored at 4°C for less than 24 h, but this should be avoided because there is a significant loss of viable organisms. Preserve tissues for histological examination in 10% neutral buffered formalin.

Intestinal and Urogenital Protozoa

Amebae. The laboratory identification of amebic infections is most commonly accomplished by the microscopic detection of organisms in stool specimens. *Entamoeba histolytica* antigens can also be detected by immunoassays, and antibody production in response to extraintestinal disease is measured by serological tests. Amebic trophozoites will not survive in unpreserved stool specimens, so specimens should be examined within 30 to 60 min of voiding. Use of preservatives is required if the examination is delayed. Extraintestinal infections are generally confirmed by serological testing, although detection of amebae in abscess material or liver biopsy samples is possible.

Ciliates. Infection with *Balantidium coli* is confirmed by the microscopic examination of voided stool specimens.

Coccidia. Detection of coccidia in stool specimens is difficult because the coccidia are small, do not stain well with traditional parasitic stains, and are shed intermittently. Examine several stool specimens. *Cryptosporidium* infections can be detected by acid-fast stains, as well as immunofluorescence and enzyme immunoassays that detect antigen in stool specimens.

Flagellates. Infections with *Giardia lamblia* can be detected by microscopic examination of stool specimens and by enzyme immunoassay and immunofluorescence. Examine several stool specimens to confirm or exclude infection. Occasionally, the string test must be used to detect trophozoites in duodenal mucus. Duodenal biopsy may also reveal

Collection and Transport

G. lamblia. Trichomonas vaginalis is responsible for some urogenital infections. Trophozoites can be observed in vaginal or prostatic secretions. Urine can be examined, but it must not be contaminated with fecal material (which can contain nonpathogenic *Trichomonas* spp.). Urine specimens must be freshly collected, because the trophozoites deteriorate rapidly. Immunofluorescence and enzyme immunoassays for antigen detection have been developed.

Microsporidia. Like coccidia, microsporidia are difficult to detect in stool specimens. Multiple specimens must be examined by microscopy.

Blood and Tissue Protozoa

Babesia **spp.** Diagnosis of babesiosis requires examination of several thick and thin smears of blood, because low-grade parasitemia is common. Serological tests have been developed, but cross-reactivity with *Plasmodium* spp. has been reported.

Leishmania **spp.** Cutaneous and visceral leishmaniasis is diagnosed by detection of amastigotes in clinical specimens or promastigotes in culture. Collect cutaneous specimens after the surface of the lesion has been disinfected with 70% alcohol. Collect samples (scrapings or biopsy specimens) from the margins of active lesions (the centers do not contain organisms). Specimens for the diagnosis of visceral leishmaniasis include spleen tissue (optimal), nasal secretions, tonsillopharyngeal mucosa, lymph node aspirates, liver biopsy samples, bone marrow, and buffy coat preparations. Prepare multiple slides for staining at the time of collection. Collect specimens for culture or animal inoculation aseptically to prevent bacterial contamination. Standardized serological tests are not commercially available. The leishmanin (Montenegro) skin test has been used, but reactivity is generally delayed until convalescence.

Plasmodium **spp.** Examine multiple blood specimens over a 36-h period, using both thick and thin smears, to confirm the diagnosis of malaria. This is especially important if the patient has been partially treated. Collect blood by finger stick, and treat the blood with either heparin or EDTA (preferred) as an anticoagulant. If blood smears are not prepared within 1 h of collection, the morphology of the infected cells will be adversely affected. Antigen detection and PCR methods have been developed but are not in common use. Serological testing is not useful for diagnosis but can confirm previous disease.

Toxoplasma gondii. Infections with *T. gondii* are confirmed by detection of the organism in biopsy specimens, buffy coat cells, or CSF or by isolation of the organism from specimens inoculated into tissue culture or laboratory animals. Because asymptomatic carriage of the organism may occur, the most reliable diagnostic tests are detection of tachyzoites in CSF or bronchoalveolar lavage fluid. Serological testing may also be helpful.

***Trypanosoma* spp.** African trypanosomiasis, caused by *T. brucei*, is diagnosed by detection of trypomastigotes in blood, lymph node and bone marrow aspirates, and CSF. Collect blood by finger stick or venipuncture, and treat the blood with EDTA. Prepare multiple thick and thin smears. Maximum parasitemia occurs during febrile episodes; if the blood is negative, examine lymph node aspirates. Immunoassays have been used to detect antigens in serum and CSF, and antibodies have been detected by serological tests. American trypanosomiasis (Chagas' disease), caused by *T. cruzi*, is diagnosed by examining thick and thin smears of blood and buffy coat cells and by examining aspirates from chagomas and enlarged lymph nodes and biopsy specimens for amastigotes and trypomastigotes. Culture of blood, aspirates, and tissues can also be performed. Serological testing can be used to confirm infections.

Intestinal Helminths

Cestodes. Diagnosis of infections with intestinal cestodes is by detection of eggs or proglottids in fecal specimens.

Nematodes. Infections with intestinal nematodes are generally confirmed by detection of the characteristic eggs in fecal specimens. The exception to this is strongyloidiasis, in which larvae are found in stool. Because detection of *Strongyloides* spp. may be difficult, examine multiple stool specimens. Special procedures for other nematodes include use of the cellulose tape technique for sampling the anal folds of patients infected with *Enterobius vermicularis*.

Trematodes. Infections with intestinal trematodes are typically confirmed by detection of eggs in fecal specimens or, in the case of *Paragonimus* spp. and some schistosomes, eggs in sputum and urine specimens, respectively. Intestinal biopsy specimens have been useful for diagnosing some parasitic infestations.

Tissue Helminths

Cestodes. The diagnosis of infections with cestodes is based on the patient's clinical presentation, history of specific travel or diet, and laboratory procedures such as serological reactivity or observation of the characteristic parasitic structures in tissue. Diagnosis of sparganosis, caused by *Spirometra* spp., is confirmed by recovery of the intact worm in the subcutaneous tissue mass or detection by histological examination of the tissue. The diagnosis of cysticercosis, caused by *Taenia solium*, and coenurosis, produced by larval *Taenia* spp., is established by recovery of cysticerci or histological demonstration of cysticerci in tissue. Hydatid disease, caused by *Echinococcus* spp., is diagnosed by radiological demonstration of cysts and serological testing. Aspiration of fluid containing "hydatid sand" is considered hazardous and should not be attempted.

Nematodes. Infections with filarial nematodes are confirmed by detection of microfilariae in blood or skin or detection of the adult worms in tissues. Adult lymphatic filariae (*Wuchereria* and *Brugia* spp.) are present in lymphatic tissues; their microfilariae migrate in the blood. *Wuchereria* microfilariae are nocturnal, and *Brugia* microfilariae are periodic. Adult *Loa loa* worms are found either in subcutaneous tissues or in the conjunctiva (eye worm); the microfilariae migrate in the blood during the daytime. Because relatively few microfilariae are present in blood, diagnosis of filariasis caused by these nematodes generally requires concentration of blood by filtration and examination of thick smears. Thin smears are usually not useful. *Onchocerca* adult worms are in fibrous subcutaneous nodules, and the microfilariae can be detected in skin and occasionally in the cornea and anterior chamber of the eye. Skin snips are obtained by biopsies of the scapular region, iliac crest, and calf. Be careful not to cause bleeding, which may confound diagnosis if blood microfilariae are present.

Collection and Transport

Mansonella species can be found in either skin tissues or blood, depending on the species. *Dracunculus* adult worms live in subcutaneous tissues and release larvae after migrating to the skin surface. Diagnosis depends on recovery of adult female worms at the surface of the skin. Diagnosis of trichinosis, caused by *Trichinella spiralis*, is confirmed by demonstrating encapsulated larvae in biopsy samples of skeletal muscle (e.g., deltoid or gastrocnemius) or serological reactivity. Nematodes associated with larva migrans are recovered by detection of eggs or larvae in tissues or by serological reactivity.

Trematodes. Most trematode infections are generally diagnosed by detection of characteristic eggs in fecal specimens. However, adult worms and occasionally eggs can be found in tissues. Identification of the worms and eggs is based on their morphologic characteristics and anatomical locations.

Collection and Transport

Collection and Transport

Table 3.1 General specimen collection and transport guidelines[a]

Specimen type	Collection		Time and temp	
	Guidelines	Device and/or minimum vol	Transport	Storage
Abscess	Remove surface exudate by wiping with sterile saline or 70% alcohol.			
Open	Aspirate fluid from deep into lesion and firmly swab, scrape, or biopsy the lesion's advancing edge.	Anaerobe transport system	≤2 h, RT	≤24 h, RT
Closed	Aspirate abscess wall material with needle and syringe. Aseptically transfer *all* material into anaerobic transport device or vial.	Anaerobic transport system, ≥1 ml	≤2 h, RT	≤24 h, RT
Bite wound	See Abscess.			
Blood culture	For disinfection of culture bottle, apply	Bacteria: blood culture, 2 bottles/set	≤2 h, RT	≤24 h, RT

70% isopropyl alcohol to rubber stoppers and wait 1 min.

For disinfection of venipuncture site:
1. Clean site with 70% alcohol.
2. Allow alcohol to dry.
3. Swab concentrically, starting at center, with iodine.
4. *Do not palpate vein at this point.*
5. Collect blood.
6. After venipuncture, remove iodine from skin with alcohol.

Adult, 20 ml/set
Child, 5–10 ml/set
Infant, 1–2 ml/set
Use the lysis-centrifugation system for intracellular or fastidious bacteria, mycobacteria, filamentous fungi, *Cryptococcus* spp.

Catheter i.v.

1. Cleanse skin around catheter site with alcohol.

Sterile screw-cap tube or cup

≤15 min, RT

≤24 h, 4°C

(continued)

Collection and Transport

Collection and Transport

Table 3.1 General specimen collection and transport guidelines[a] (continued)

	Collection		Time and temp	
Specimen type	Guidelines	Device and/or minimum vol	Transport	Storage
	2. Remove catheter aseptically; clip 5-cm distal tip and catheter segment that passes through the skin surface. Place in sterile tube or cup. Transport directly to microbiology laboratory to prevent drying.			
Foley	Do *not* culture, since growth represents distal urethral flora.			
Cellulitis	1. Clean skin by wiping with sterile saline or 70% alcohol. 2. Aspirate area of maximum	Sterile screw-cap tube	≤15 min, RT	≤24 h, 4°C

	inflammation with fine needle and syringe.		
	3. Draw small amount of sterile saline into syringe.		
	4. Inject into a sterile tube.		
CSF	1. Disinfect site with iodine.	Sterile screw-cap tube Bacteria, ≥1 ml Fungi, ≥2 ml AFB, ≥2 ml Virus, ≥1 ml	Bacteria: ≤15 min, RT (never refrigerate) Viruses: ≤15 min, 4°C (send on ice)	≤2 h, RT ≤72 h, 4°C
	2. Insert needle with stylet at L3-L4, L4-L5, or L5-S1 interspace.		
	3. Upon reaching subarachnoid space, remove stylet, and collect at least 1 ml of fluid into each of three leakproof tubes.		
Decubitus ulcer	1. Cleanse surface with sterile saline.	Swab transport or anaerobic system	≤2 h, RT	≤24 h, RT

(continued)

Collection and Transport

Table 3.1 General specimen collection and transport guidelines*a* (*continued*)

Specimen type	Collection			Time and temp	
	Guidelines	Device and/or minimum vol		Transport	Storage
	2. If biopsy sample is not available, *vigorously* swab base of lesion. Do not collect superficial exudate. 3. Place swab or biopsy specimen into an appropriate transport system.	(anaerobe cultures of very limited value)			
Dental culture: gingival, periodontal, periapical, Vincent's stomatitis	1. Carefully clean gingival margin and supragingival tooth surface to remove saliva, debris, and plaque. 2. Using periodontal scaler, carefully remove subgingival lesion material and	Anaerobic transport system		≤2 h, RT	≤24 h, RT

	transfer it to anaerobic transport system.		
Ear Inner	Tympanocentesis is reserved for complicated, recurrent, or chronic otitis media.	Anaerobic system	≤2 h, RT
	1. For intact ear drum, clean ear canal with soap solution, dry, and collect fluid via syringe aspiration technique.		≤2 h, RT
	2. For ruptured ear drum, collect fluid on flexible-shaft swab via auditory speculum.		
Outer	1. Use moistened swab to remove any debris or crust from ear canal.	Swab transport or anaerobic system	≤24 h, RT
	2. Obtain sample by firmly rotating swab in outer canal.		

(continued)

Collection and Transport

Collection and Transport

Table 3.1 General specimen collection and transport guidelines[a] (*continued*)

| Specimen type | Collection | | | Time and temp | |
	Guidelines	Device and/or minimum vol		Transport	Storage
	3. Biopsy if deep involvement.				
Eye					
Conjunctiva	1. Sample both eyes with separate swabs (premoistened with sterile saline) by rolling swab over each conjunctiva. 2. Inoculate medium at time of collection. 3. Smear swabs onto two slides for staining.	Direct culture inoculation		Plates: ≤15 min, RT	≤2 h, RT
Corneal scrapings	1. Obtain conjunctival swab specimens as described above. 2. Instill 2 drops of local anesthetic.	Direct culture inoculation		≤15 min, RT	≤2 h, RT

	3. Using sterile spatula, scrape ulcers or lesions, and inoculate scraping directly onto medium. 4. Apply remaining material to two clean glass slides for staining.		
Feces			
Routine culture	Pass directly into clean, dry container. Transport to microbiology laboratory within 1 h of collection, or transfer to enteric transport system.	Sterile, leakproof, wide-mouth container or enteric transport system, ≥2 g	≤24 h, 4°C Enteric transport system: ≤48 h, RT
		Unpreserved: ≤1 h, RT	
Clostridium difficile	Perform toxin assay with liquid or soft stool passed directly into clean, dry container. Soft stool is defined as stool that assumes	Sterile, leakproof, wide-mouth container, ≥5 ml	3 days, 4°C; >3 days, −70°C
		≤1 h, RT	

(continued)

Collection and Transport

Table 3.1 General specimen collection and transport guidelines[a] *(continued)*

| Specimen type | Collection | | Time and temp | |
	Guidelines	Device and/or minimum vol	Transport	Storage
	the shape of its container. Dry, formed stools should not be processed.			
Escherichia coli O157:H7	Pass liquid and/or bloody stool into clean, dry container.	Sterile, leakproof, wide-mouth container or enteric transport system, >2 ml	Unpreserved: ≤1 h, RT	≤24 h, 4°C Enteric transport system: ≤48 h, RT
Rectal swab	1. Carefully insert swab ≈1 in. beyond anal sphincter. 2. Gently rotate swab to sample anal crypts.	Swab transport	≤1 h, RT	≤24 h, RT
Fistula	See Abscess.			
Fluid: abdominal, ascites, bile, joint, pericardial, peritoneal, pleural, synovial	1. Disinfect overlying skin with iodine. 2. Obtain specimen via percutaneous needle aspiration or surgery.	Sterile screw-cap tube or anaerobic transport system, ≥1 ml; specimens for bacterial/fungal culture	≤15 min, RT	≤2 h, RT, except pericardial fluid and fungal cultures

	3. Transport immediately to laboratory. 4. Always submit as much fluid as possible; *never* submit swab dipped in fluid.	should be inoculated directly into blood culture bottles.
Gangrenous tissue	See Abscess.	
Gastric wash or lavage fluid	Collect in early morning before patients eat and while they are still in bed. 1. Introduce nasogastric tube orally or nasally to stomach. 2. Perform lavage with 25–50 ml of chilled, sterile, distilled water. 3. Recover sample and place in leakproof sterile container. 4. Before removing tube, release suction and clamp it.	Sterile leakproof container ≤15 min, RT, or neutralize with sodium carbonate within 1 h of collection ≤24 h, 4°C

(continued)

Table 3.1 General specimen collection and transport guidelines[a] (continued)

| Specimen type | Collection | | Time and temp | |
	Guidelines	Device and/or minimum vol	Transport	Storage
Genital: female				
Amniotic	1. Aspirate via amniocentesis, cesarean section, or intrauterine catheter. 2. Transfer fluid to anaerobic transport system.	Anaerobic transport system, ≥1 ml	≤15 min, RT	≤24 h, RT
Bartholin	See Abscess.			
Cervix	1. Visualize cervix with speculum without lubricant. 2. Remove mucus and/or secretions from cervix with swab, and discard swab. 3. Firmly yet gently, sample endocervical canal with sterile swab.	Anaerobic transport system	≤2 h, RT	≤24 h, RT

Collection and Transport

Cul-de-sac	Submit aspirate or fluid.	Anaerobic transport system, >1 ml	≤2 h, RT	≤24 h, RT
Endometrium	1. Collect transcervical aspirate via telescoping catheter. 2. Transfer entire amount to anaerobic transport system.	Anaerobic transport system, ≥1 ml	≤2 h, RT	≤24 h, RT
Products of conception	1. Submit portion of tissue in sterile container. 2. If obtained by cesarean section, immediately transfer to anaerobic transport system.	Sterile tube or anaerobic transport system	≤2 h, RT	≤24 h, RT
Urethra	1. Remove exudate from urethral orifice. 2. Collect discharge material on swab by massaging urethra against pubic symphysis through vagina.	Swab transport	≤2 h, RT	≤24 h, RT

(continued)

Collection and Transport

Collection and Transport

Table 3.1 General specimen collection and transport guidelines[a] *(continued)*

| Specimen type | Collection | | Time and temp | |
	Guidelines	Device and/or minimum vol	Transport	Storage
Vagina	1. Wipe away excessive amount of secretion or discharge. 2. Obtain secretions from mucosal membrane of vaginal vault with sterile swab. 3. If smear is also requested, obtain it with second swab.	Swab transport	≤2 h, RT	≤24 h, RT
Genital: female or male				
Lesion	1. Clean lesion with sterile saline, and remove surface of lesion with sterile scalpel blade. 2. Allow transudate to accumulate.	Swab transport	≤2 h, RT	≤24 h, RT

	3. While pressing base of lesion, *firmly* sample exudate with sterile swab.			
Genital: male				
Prostate	1. Clean glans with soap and water. 2. Massage prostate through rectum. 3. Collect fluid on sterile swab or in sterile tube.	Swab transport or sterile tube	≤2 h, RT	≤24 h, RT
Urethra	Insert urethrogenital swab ≈1 in. into urethral lumen, rotate swab, and leave it in place for at least 2 s.	Swab transport	≤2 h, RT	≤24 h, RT
Hair: dermatophytosis	1. With forceps, collect at least 10–12 affected hairs with bases of shafts intact. 2. Place in clean tube or container.	Clean container, 10 hairs	≤24 h, RT	≤24 h, RT

(continued)

Collection and Transport

Table 3.1 General specimen collection and transport guidelines[a] *(continued)*

	Collection		Time and temp	
Specimen type	Guidelines	Device and/or minimum vol	Transport	Storage
Nail: dermatophytosis	1. Wipe nail with 70% alcohol. Use gauze (not cotton). 2. Clip away generous portion of affected area, and collect material or debris from under nail. 3. Place material in clean container.	Clean container, enough scrapings to cover head of thumbtack	≤24 h, RT	≤24 h, RT
Pilonidal cyst	See Abscess.			
Respiratory tract, lower BAL, BW, BB, tracheal aspirate	1. Place aspirate or washing into sputum trap. 2. Place brush in sterile container with saline.	Sterile container: Bacteria, 1 ml; fungi, ≥2 ml; mycobacteria, ≥2 ml; viruses, ≥1 ml	≤2 h, RT	≤24 h, 4°C

Sputum, expectorate	1. Collect specimen under *direct* supervision of nurse or physician. 2. Have patient rinse or gargle with water. 3. Instruct patient to cough *deeply* to produce lower respiratory specimen (not postnasal fluid). Collect into sterile container.	Sterile container: as above	≤2 h, RT	≤24 h, 4°C
Sputum, induced	1. Have patient rinse mouth with water after brushing gums and tongue. 2. With aid of nebulizer, have patient inhale ≈25 ml of 3–10% sterile saline. 3. Collect induced sputum into sterile container.	Sterile container: as above	≤2 h, RT	≤24 h, 4°C

Collection and Transport

(continued)

Collection and Transport

Table 3.1 General specimen collection and transport guidelines[a] *(continued)*

| Specimen type | Collection | | Time and temp | |
	Guidelines	Device and/or minimum vol	Transport	Storage
Respiratory tract, upper				
Oral	1. Remove oral secretions or debris from surface of lesion with swab, and discard swab. 2. Using second swab, vigorously sample lesion, avoiding saliva and any areas of normal tissue.	Swab transport	≤2 h, RT	≤24 h, RT
Nasal	1. Use swab premoistened with sterile saline. Insert ≈1 in. into nares. 2. Rotate swab against nasal mucosa.	Swab transport	≤2 h, RT	≤24 h, RT
Nasopharynx	1. Gently insert calcium alginate swab into posterior nasopharynx via nose.	Direct medium inoculation or swab transport	Plates: ≤15 min, RT Swabs: ≤2 h, RT	≤24 h, RT

	Procedure	Container	Transport
	2. Rotate swab slowly for 5 s to absorb secretions. Remove swab; inoculate medium at bedside, or place swab in transport medium.	Swab transport	≤24 h, RT
Throat	1. Depress tongue with tongue depressor. 2. Sample posterior pharynx, tonsils, and inflamed areas with sterile swab.	Swab transport	≤2 h, RT
Skin: dermatophytosis	1. Cleanse affected area with 70% alcohol. 2. Gently scrape surface of skin at *active margin* of lesion. *Do not draw blood.* 3. Place sample in clean container.	Clean container, enough scrapings to cover head of thumbtack	≤24 h, RT
Tissue	1. Submit in sterile container.	Anaerobic transport system	≤15 min, RT ≤24 h, RT

(continued)

Collection and Transport

Table 3.1 General specimen collection and transport guidelines[a] (*continued*)

| Specimen type | Collection | | Time and temp | |
	Guidelines	Device and/or minimum vol	Transport	Storage
	2. For small samples, add several drops of sterile saline to keep moist.			
	3. *Do not allow tissue to dry out.*			
	4. Place in anaerobic transport system.			
Urine				
Female, midstream	1. Thoroughly clean urethral area with soap and water.	Sterile wide-mouth container, ≥1 ml, or urine transport kit	Unpreserved: ≤2 h, RT	≤24 h, 4°C Preserved: ≤24 h, RT
	2. Rinse area with wet gauze pads.			
	3. While holding labia apart, begin voiding.			

	4. Collect the first-voided specimen for gonorrhea and chlamydia testing if required. 5. After passage of several milliliters, collect midstream portion without stopping flow of urine.		
Male, midstream	1. Clean the glans with soap and water. 2. Rinse area with wet gauze pads. 3. While holding foreskin retracted, begin voiding. 4. Collect first-voided specimen and midstream specimen as described above.	Sterile wide-mouth container, ≥1 ml, or urine transport kit	Unpreserved: ≤2 h, RT ≤24 h, 4°C Preserved: ≤24 h, RT
Wound	See Abscess.		

^{a}AFB, acid-fast bacilli; BAL, bronchoalveolar lavage; BB, bronchial brushing; BW, bronchial washing; RT, room temperature.

Collection and Transport

Table 3.2 Confirmation of food-borne infectious disease outbreaks[a]

Etiologic agent	Specimen and tests
Bacterial	
Bacillus cereus	Isolation of organism from stool of two or more ill persons and not from stool of controls; *or* isolation of $\geq 10^5$ organisms/g from epidemiologically implicated food
Brucella spp.	Isolation of organism from two or more ill persons; *or* positive serological test (fourfold increase in agglutination titers or single titer $\geq 1:160$) in patients with compatible clinical symptoms and history of exposure
Campylobacter spp.	Isolation of organism from two or more ill persons; or isolation of organism from epidemiologically implicated food
Clostridium botulinum	Detection of botulinal toxin in serum, stool, gastric contents, or implicated food; *or* isolation of organism from stool or intestine
Clostridium perfringens	Isolation of $\geq 10^6$ organism/g in stool of two or more ill persons; *or* demonstration of enterotoxin in the stool of two or more ill persons; *or* isolation of $\geq 10^5$ organisms/g from epidemiologically implicated food
Escherichia coli	
Enterohemorrhagic	Isolation of *E. coli* O157:H7 or other Shiga-like toxin-producing *E. coli* from two or more ill persons; *or* isolation of *E. coli* O157:H7 or other Shiga-like toxin-producing *E. coli* from implicated food

Enterotoxigenic	Isolation of organism of same serotype, producing heat-stable or heat-labile enterotoxins, from stool of two or more ill persons
Enteropathogenic	Isolation of organism of same serotype from stool of two or more ill persons
Enteroinvasive	Isolation of same enteroinvasive serotype from stool of two or more ill persons
Listeria monocytogenes	Isolation of organism of same serotype from stool of two or more ill persons exposed to food that is epidemiologically implicated or from which organism of same serotype has been isolated
Salmonella typhi	Isolation of organisms from clinical specimens of two or more ill persons; *or* isolation of organisms from epidemiologically implicated food
Salmonella s nontyphoidal	Isolation of organism from clinical specimens of two or more ill persons; *or* isolation of organism from epidemiologically implicated food
Shigella spp.	Isolation of organisms of same serotype from clinical specimens from two or more ill persons; *or* isolation of organism from epidemiologically implicated food
Staphylococcus aureus	Isolation of organism of same phage type from stool or vomitus of two or more ill persons; *or* detection of enterotoxin in epidemiologically implicated food; *or* isolation of $\geq 10^5$ organisms/g from epidemiologically implicated food
Streptococcus group A	Isolation of organism of same M or T type from throats of two or more ill persons; *or* isolation of organism of same M or T type from implicated food

(continued)

Collection and Transport

Collection and Transport

Table 3.2 Confirmation of food-borne infectious disease outbreaks[a] *(continued)*

Etiologic agent	Specimen and tests
Vibrio cholerae, O1 or O139	Isolation of toxigenic organism from stool or vomitus of two or more ill persons; *or* significant rise in vibriocidal, bacterial agglutinating, or antitoxin antibodies; *or* isolation of organism from epidemiologically implicated food
Vibrio cholerae, other serotypes	Isolation of organism of same serotype from stool of two or more ill persons
Vibrio parahaemolyticus	Isolation of Kanagawa-positive organism from stool of two or more ill persons; *or* isolation of $\geq 10^5$ Kanagawa-positive organisms/g from epidemiologically implicated food provided specimen was properly handled
Yersinia enterocolitica	Isolation of organism from clinical specimen of two or more ill persons; *or* isolation of pathogenic strain of organisms from epidemiologically implicated food
Parasitic	
Cryptosporidium parvum	Demonstration of organism or antigen in stool or in small bowel biopsy specimen of two or more ill persons; *or* demonstration of organism in epidemiologically implicated food
Cyclospora cayetanensis	Demonstration of organism in stool of two or more ill persons

Organism	Criteria
Giardia lamblia	Detection of antigen in stool of two or more ill persons; *or* demonstration of organism in stool, duodenal contents, or small bowel biopsy specimen in stool of two or more ill persons
Trichinella spp.	Positive serological test in two or more ill persons; *or* demonstration of larvae in muscle biopsy specimen of two or more ill persons; *or* demonstration of larvae in epidemiologically implicated meat
Viral	
Hepatitis A virus	Detection of IgM anti-hepatitis A virus in serum from two or more persons who consumed epidemiologically implicated food
Norwalk and Norwalk-like viruses	Fourfold or greater rise in antibody titer to viruses; *or* demonstration of small, round viruses that react by immune electron microscopy; *or* detection of virus by molecular diagnostics in two or more ill patients
Astrovirus, calicivirus, and others	Detection of small, round viruses that react by immune electron microscopy; *or* detection of virus by molecular diagnostics in two or more ill patients

[a]Modified from *Morbid. Mortal. Weekly Rep.* **45** (SS-5):59–66, 1996.

Collection and Transport

Specimen Processing

This section provides general guidelines for processing specimens for microbiology tests. Testing can be subdivided into microscopy, culture, antigen tests (including immunoassay and molecular diagnostic tests), and antibody tests. Although it is impossible to provide guidelines for all possible infections, the most common organisms associated with human disease are included. Interpretive criteria for antigen and antibody tests are discussed in greater detail in section 7, Immunodiagnostic Tests.

Primary Plating Media: Bacteria

Bacteroides Bile-Esculin (BBE) Agar

Bacteroides bile-esculin agar is a selective, differential agar medium used for the recovery of the *Bacteroides fragilis* group. The medium contains oxgall (bile), esculin, ferric ammonium citrate, hemin, vitamin K_1, and gentamicin in a casein and soybean agar base. Growth of non-*B. fragilis* group organisms is inhibited by the bile and the gentamicin. Supplementation of the agar with hemin and vitamin K_1 stimulates the growth of *Bacteroides* spp. Esculin hydrolysis is detected when esculin is converted to esculetin and reacts with ferric ammonium citrate to produce black colonies.

Bile-Esculin (Enterococcal Selective) Agar

Bile-esculin agar can be made selective for the recovery of vancomycin-resistant enterococci by adding 6 μg of vancomycin per ml to it. Enterococci are able to grow in the presence of bile and hydrolyze esculin. Vancomycin-resistant strains produce black colonies on this agar, but susceptible strains fail to grow.

Bismuth Sulfite Agar

Bismuth sulfite agar is a differential, selective medium used for the isolation and identification of *Salmonella typhi* and other enteric bacilli. The medium contains digests of casein and animal tissue, beef extract, glucose, ferric sulfate, and bismuth sulfite. Most commensal organisms are inhibited by the bismuth sulfite. *S. typhi* colonies appear black with a metallic sheen.

Blood Agar

Many types of blood agar media are used in clinical laboratories. The two basic components are the basal medium (e.g., brain heart infusion, brucella, Columbia, Schaedler's, tryptic soy) and blood (e.g., sheep, horse, rabbit). Additional supplements are commonly used to enhance the growth of specific organisms or to suppress the growth of unwanted organisms.

Bordet-Gengou Agar

Recovery of *Bordetella pertussis* and *Bordetella parapertussis* is inhibited by factors such as fatty acids, metal ions, sulfides, and peroxides that are commonly present in media. Starch, charcoal, serum albumin, blood, or similar components are added to the medium to neutralize these inhibitors. Bordet-Gengou agar is a potato infusion-glycerol-based agar medium supplemented with 20 to 30% sheep, horse, or rabbit blood. Potato infusion is required for the growth of *Bordetella* spp., and glycerol is added to conserve moisture in the medium. Antibiotics such as methicillin or cephalexin are commonly added to suppress the growth of bacteria such as staphylococci, which inhibit the growth of *Bordetella* spp. Because this medium must be made fresh (it has a shelf life of less than 1 week), it has largely been replaced by Regan-Lowe agar.

Brilliant Green Agar

Brilliant green agar is a selective, differential medium for the recovery of *Salmonella* spp. The medium contains digests of casein and animal tissues, lactose, sucrose, phenol red, and brilliant green. *Salmonella* spp. appear as red, pink, or white colonies surrounded by a red zone, indicating their inability to ferment lactose or sucrose. Lactose- or sucrose-fermenting bacteria that grow on this medium form yellow-green colonies surrounded by a zone of yellow-green.

Buffered Charcoal-Yeast Extract (BCYE) Agar

Buffered charcoal-yeast extract agar is selective for the recovery of *Legionella* and *Nocardia* spp. It contains agar, yeast extract, charcoal, and salts and is supplemented with L-cysteine, ferric pyrophosphate, ACES [*N*-(2-acetamido)-2-aminoethanesulfonic acid] buffer, and α-ketoglutarate. The charcoal detoxifies the medium, the yeast extracts are rich in nutrients, and the L-cysteine, ferric pyrophosphate, and α-ketoglutarate stimulate the growth of *Legionella* spp. The addition of ACES is required to buffer the medium because *Legionella* spp. have a narrow pH tolerance (growth is optimal at pH 6.9). Various antibiotics such as polymyxin B, anisomycin, cefamandole, vancomycin, and cycloheximide are added to inhibit the growth of other bacteria when nonsterile clinical and environmental specimens are cultured.

Campylobacter Selective Medium

A large number of media have been developed for the selective isolation of *Campylobacter* spp. from stool specimens. Most use a brucella basal medium, which preferentially supports the growth of *Campylobacter* spp. Blood is added, as are various combinations of antibiotics (e.g., cephalothin, vancomycin, trimethoprim, amphotericin, and polymyxin in the Blaser-Wang formulation; cycloheximide, cefazolin, novobiocin, bacitracin, and colistin in the Butzler formulation; cycloheximide, cefoperazone, and vancomycin in the Karmali formulation; and cycloheximide rifampin, trimethoprim, and polymyxin in the Preston formulation).

Cefsulodin-Irgasan-Novobiocin (CIN) Agar

Cefsulodin-Irgasan-novobiocin agar is a selective, differential agar medium used for the isolation of *Yersinia* and *Aeromonas* spp. The medium consists of digests of animal tissue and gelatin, beef and yeast extracts, sodium pyruvate, sodium deoxycholate, neutral red, crystal violet, cefsulodin, Irgasan, and novobiocin. The antibiotics and sodium deoxycholate inhibit the growth of most organisms in stool specimens. However, *Yersinia* and *Aeromonas* spp. are resistant and can ferment mannitol in the medium. This fermentation produces colonies with a bull's eye appearance, i.e., deep red centers with transparent edges.

Chocolate Agar

Chocolate agar is an enriched medium that derives its name from its color. Blood or hemoglobin is added immediately after the medium is heated, and the heat causes the added component to lyse and turn brown. This medium supports the growth of most bacteria and is required for the recovery of many species of *Haemophilus* and some pathogenic strains of *Neisseria*. A variety of formulations of this medium have been used, but the most common consists of a peptone base enriched with 2% hemoglobin or IsoVitaleX. Catalase-negative bacteria (e.g., *Streptococcus pneu-*

moniae) grow less well on this medium than on blood agar because catalase from ruptured erythrocytes in blood agar is not available to protect the bacteria from peroxides that accumulate in the medium.

Chopped-Meat Broth

Chopped-meat broth is an enriched broth used for the recovery of a variety of bacteria, particularly anaerobes, from clinical specimens. Extracts as well as solid particles of beef or horse meat are suspended in broth with peptones, yeast extract sugars, starch, and L-cysteine. The L-cysteine helps maintain a low E_h (oxidation-reduction potential), which supports the growth of anaerobes.

Colistin-Nalidixic Acid (CNA) Agar

Colistin-nalidixic acid agar is a selective medium used for the recovery of aerobic and anaerobic gram-positive bacteria. The medium consists of Columbia agar base supplemented with nalidixic acid, colistin, and blood. Nalidixic acid inhibits most aerobic gram-negative bacilli, as does colistin. The *B. fragilis* group is usually resistant to these antibiotics, but other anaerobic gram-negative bacilli can be inhibited by colistin.

Cycloserine-Cefoxitin-Egg Yolk-Fructose Agar (CCFA)

Cycloserine-cefoxitin-egg yolk-fructose agar is a selective, differential medium used for the recovery of *Clostridium difficile*. The medium consists of animal tissue digest, fructose, cycloserine, cefoxitin, and neutral red. Cycloserine and cefoxitin inhibit most intestinal bacteria. *C. difficile* can ferment fructose, producing a more acidic pH, which is detected by the indicator dye neutral red (shift from red to yellow medium surrounding the colonies). Various modifications of this medium are used, including supplementation with egg yolk to stimulate growth of clostridia.

Cystine Lactose Electrolyte-Deficient (CLED) Agar

Cystine lactose electrolyte-deficient agar is a nonselective differential medium used for the recovery of urinary tract pathogens. The medium consists of casein and gelatin digests, beef extract, L-cystine, lactose, and bromthymol blue. Lactose-fermenting bacteria have yellow colonies, and the swarming of motile gram-negative bacilli is inhibited.

Cystine Tellurite Blood Agar

Cystine tellurite blood agar medium is a selective, differential medium used for the recovery of *Corynebacterium diphtheriae*. The medium consists of heart infusion agar, potassium tellurite, L-cystine, and rabbit blood. Potassium tellurite inhibits the growth of most commensal organisms and allows *C. diphtheriae* to grow. The organism produces hydrogen sulfide from cystine, and the reaction of tellurite with hydrogen sulfide results in brown halos surrounding the colonies of *C. diphtheriae*.

Ellinghausen & McCullough Modified Bovine Albumin Tween 80 Medium

The modified bovine albumin Tween 80 medium is selective for the growth of leptospiras. The basal medium, consisting of glycerol, sodium pyruvate, and thiamine, is supplemented with bovine albumin, Tween 80, vitamin B_{12}, and salts of iron, calcium, magnesium, zinc, and copper.

Eosin-Methylene Blue (EMB) Agar

Eosin-methylene blue agar is a differential, selective medium used for the isolation and differentiation of lactose-fermenting and -nonfermenting gram-negative bacilli. The agar medium consists of casein digests, lactose, sucrose, eosin Y, and methylene blue. The Levine formulation does not include sucrose. Growth of gram-positive bacteria is suppressed by the methylene blue, which, together with eosin Y, also serves as an indicator for carbohydrate fermentation (dyes precipitate at an acidic pH). Bacteria that ferment lactose (e.g., *Escherichia*, *Klebsiella*, and *Enterobacter* spp.) have colonies with a green metallic sheen or that are blue-black to brown. Nonfermentative bacteria (e.g., *Proteus*, *Salmonella*, and *Shigella* spp.) have colorless or light purple colonies.

Fletcher Medium

Fletcher medium is a semisolid medium used for the recovery of *Leptospira* spp. The medium consists of 0.15% agar, salt, peptones, beef extract, and rabbit serum. *Leptospira* spp. usually grow within 1 to 2 weeks in this medium.

Gram-Negative (GN; Hajna) Broth

Gram-negative broth is a selective enrichment broth used for the recovery of small numbers of salmonellae and shigellae from stool specimens. The medium consists of digests of casein and animal tissues, mannitol, glucose, sodium citrate, and sodium deoxycholate. The sodium citrate and sodium deoxycholate inhibit the growth of many gram-positive and gram-negative bacteria. The fact that the concentration of mannitol is higher than that of glucose limits the growth of *Proteus* spp. However, commensal organisms will overgrow the enteric pathogens if the broth is incubated for more than 4 to 6 h.

Hektoen Enteric (HE) Agar

Hektoen enteric agar is a selective medium used for the isolation of *Salmonella* and *Shigella* spp. and differentiation of these organisms from other gram-negative bacilli that may be recovered on this medium. It consists of a peptone base agar supplemented with bile salts, lactose, sucrose, salicin, ferric ammonium citrate, and the pH indicators bromthymol blue and acid fuchsin. The bile inhibits all gram-positive bacteria and many gram-negative bacilli. Acids produced by fermentation of lactose, sucrose, or salicin react with bromthymol blue to produce a yellow color and with acid fuchsin to produce a red color. Hydrogen sulfide produced by the metabolism of sodium thiosulfate is detected when a black precipitate forms after the addition of ferric ammonium citrate. Lactose-fermenting bacteria (e.g., *Escherichia coli*) are slightly inhibited on this agar and appear as orange or salmon pink colonies. *Salmonella* colonies typically appear blue-green with black centers. *Shigella* colonies appear green with no black center. *Proteus* spp. are inhibited; their colonies are colorless.

Kanamycin-Vancomycin Laked Blood (LKV) Agar

Kanamycin-vancomycin laked blood agar is a selective, differential medium used for the recovery of anaerobic gram-negative bacilli, especially *Bacteroides* and *Prevotella* spp. The medium consists of casein and soybean meal agar supplemented with kanamycin, vancomycin, vitamin K_1, and lysed (laked) sheep blood. Kanamycin inhibits most facultative, gram-negative bacilli, and vancomycin inhibits most gram-positive organisms and *Porphyromonas* spp. Vitamin K_1 stimulates the growth of some *Prevotella* strains, which also will develop a black pigment in the presence of lysed blood.

Kelly Medium

Kelly medium is used for the isolation of *Borrelia* species from human specimens and arthropod vectors. The success of these cultures depends on the quality of the medium. In general, specimens should be submitted to reference laboratories for processing. A modified version (Barbour-Stoenner-Kelly II medium) of the original formulation is currently used. The medium consists of peptone and casein digests, albumin, gelatin, rabbit serum, hemin, yeast extracts, glucose, and a complex mixture of buffers, amino acids, vitamins, nucleotides, and other growth factors. Kanamycin and 5-fluorouracil have been added to the medium for the selective isolation of borreliae from contaminated specimens. Recovery of the organisms requires prolonged incubation in a microaerophilic atmosphere at 30 to 37°C. Organisms are detected by examining the broth at weekly intervals by dark-field microscopy.

LIM Broth

LIM broth is a selective enrichment broth used for the recovery of group B streptococci. The medium consists of Todd-Hewitt broth supplemented with yeast extract, colistin, and nalidixic acid. Most aerobic and anaerobic gram-negative bacilli are inhibited by the antibiotics, while group B streptococci grow well in this broth.

Loeffler Medium

Loeffler medium is an enriched medium used for the recovery of *Corynebacterium diphtheriae*. The medium consists of animal digests, heart muscle infusion, beef serum, egg, and glucose. *C. diphtheriae* grows rapidly on this medium, and Gram stains of colonies demonstrate characteristic metachromatic granules.

MacConkey (MAC) Agar

MacConkey agar is a selective agar medium used for the isolation and differentiation of lactose-fermenting and -nonfermenting gram-negative bacilli. The medium consists of digests of peptones, bile salts, lactose, neutral red, and crystal violet. Bile salts and crystal violet inhibit the growth of gram-positive bacteria and some fastidious gram-negative bacteria. Colonies that ferment lactose (e.g., *Escherichia*, *Klebsiella*, and *Enterobacter* spp.) produce acid, which causes a red color shift in the neutral red pH indicator and precipitates the bile salts. Colonies appear red to pink, while nonfermenting colonies (e.g., *Proteus*, *Salmonella*, and *Shigella* spp.) appear yellow, colorless, or translucent.

Mannitol Salt Agar
Mannitol salt agar is a selective medium used for the isolation of staphylococci. The medium consists of digests of casein and animal tissue, beef extract, mannitol, salt, and phenol red indicator. If the organism can grow in the presence of 7.5% salt and ferment mannitol, the acid turns the indicator yellow. Most strains of *Staphylococcus aureus* produce yellow colonies, while coagulase-negative staphylococci do not ferment the mannitol and thus remain red. Most other organisms are inhibited by the high salt concentration.

New York City Agar
New York City agar is a selective medium used for the isolation of pathogenic *Neisseria* spp. The medium consists of peptones, cornstarch, yeast dialysate, glucose, hemoglobin, horse plasma, and a mixture of antibiotics (vancomycin, colistin, amphotericin B, and trimethoprim). This medium can be used instead of Thayer-Martin agar.

Phenylethyl Alcohol (PEA) Blood Agar
Phenylethyl alcohol blood agar is a selective medium that consists of casein and soybean agar supplemented with phenylethyl alcohol and blood. Facultative gram-negative bacilli are inhibited by the phenylethyl alcohol (e.g., the growth of swarming *Proteus* spp. is suppressed). Most gram-positive and gram-negative anaerobes, as well as aerobic gram-positive bacteria, will grow on this medium. *Pseudomonas* spp. are not inhibited on this medium.

Pseudomonas cepacia (PC) Agar
PC agar is a selective, differential medium used for the isolation of *Burkholderia* (*Pseudomonas*) *cepacia* from clinical specimens contaminated with other organisms. The medium consists of salt solutions, phosphate buffer, pyruvate, proteose peptones, bile, crystal violet, ticarcillin, polymyxin B, and phenol red. *Burkholderia* spp. are able to grow on this medium and metabolize pyruvate, producing alkaline by-products. Pink to red colonies are observed

after 2 days of incubation. Other bacteria are inhibited by the crystal violet and antibiotics.

Regan-Lowe Agar Medium

Regan-Lowe agar medium, for the selective isolation of *Bordetella* spp., contains beef extract, gelatin digest, starch, charcoal, niacin, 10% horse blood, and cephalexin (40 µg/ml). The charcoal and horse blood are required to neutralize fatty acids and other inhibitory factors present in the medium. Sheep but not human blood can replace horse blood. Cephalexin can delay the detection of *Bordetella* spp. on this medium, but the use of an additional nonselective medium is not considered necessary. The shelf life of this medium is 6 to 8 weeks.

Salmonella-Shigella (SS) Agar

Salmonella-shigella agar is a highly selective medium for the recovery of *Salmonella* and *Shigella* spp. The medium consists of beef extract and peptone digests, lactose as a carbohydrate source, bile salts, sodium citrate, sodium thiosulfate, neutral red, brilliant green, and ferric citrate. Bile salts, sodium citrate, and brilliant green are inhibitory for all gram-positive and selected gram-negative bacteria. Bacteria that grow on the medium and produce hydrogen sulfide from the metabolism of sodium thiosulfate are detected by the black precipitate formed with ferric citrate. Acid produced from lactose fermentation is detected with the pH indicator neutral red. All lactose-fermenting bacteria form pink or red colonies, while nonfermenting bacteria form either colorless (e.g., *Shigella* spp.) or black (e.g., *Salmonella* spp.) colonies.

Selenite Broth

Selenite broth is a selective enrichment broth used for the isolation of *Salmonella* spp. from stools and other contaminated specimens. It consists of peptones, sodium phosphate, lactose, and sodium selenite. *E. coli* and other gram-negative bacilli are inhibited by sodium selenite. The broth should be subcultured within 8 to 12 h after inoculation with the specimen, or else the enteric pathogens will be overgrown with commensal organisms.

Sorbitol-MacConkey Agar

Sorbitol-MacConkey agar is a selective differential agar used for the isolation of *E. coli* O157. Lactose is replaced with sorbitol. Most *E. coli* strains ferment sorbitol; however, *E. coli* O157 does not, and therefore its colonies are colorless on this agar.

Tetrathionate Broth

Tetrathionate broth is a selective enrichment broth used for the recovery of *Salmonella* spp. from stool specimens. It consists of a peptone base supplemented with yeast extract, mannitol, glucose, sodium deoxycholate, sodium thiosulfate, calcium carbonate, and brilliant green. The sodium deoxycholate, sodium thiosulfate, and brilliant green inhibit gram-positive and gram-negative bacteria. The broth should be subcultured 12 to 24 h after inoculation to prevent overgrowth of *Salmonella* spp. with commensal organisms.

Thayer-Martin (Modified) Agar

Many modifications of Thayer-Martin medium have been developed for the isolation of pathogenic *Neisseria* spp. The blood agar base medium is enriched with hemoglobin and supplements. The growth of unwanted bacteria can be suppressed by the addition of antibiotics such as colistin (which inhibits most gram-negative bacteria except *Proteus* spp.), trimethoprim (which inhibits *Proteus* spp.), vancomycin (which inhibits most gram-positive bacteria), and nystatin (which inhibits yeasts). Some strains of *Neisseria gonorrhoeae* are inhibited by vancomycin, so nonselective media (e.g., chocolate agar) should be used for primary isolation.

Thioglycolate Broth

Thioglycolate broth is an enrichment broth used for the recovery of aerobic and anaerobic bacteria. Various formulations are used, but most include casein digest, glucose, yeast extract, cysteine, and sodium thioglycolate. Supplementation with hemin and vitamin K_1 will enhance the recovery of anaerobic bacteria.

Thiosulfate Citrate Bile Salts Sucrose (TCBS) Agar

Thiosulfate citrate bile salts sucrose agar is a selective, differential medium used for the recovery of *Vibrio* spp. The medium consists of digests of casein and animal tissue, yeast extract, sodium citrate, sodium cholate, oxgall (bile), sucrose, ferric citrate, thymol blue, and bromthymol blue. Sodium citrate, sodium cholate, and bile inhibit commensal organisms. *Vibrio cholerae* colonies are yellow on this medium due to fermentation of sucrose with the acid, resulting in a yellow color shift of the indicator, bromthymol blue. *Vibrio parahaemolyticus* fails to ferment sucrose, and the colonies are therefore blue-green. Some enteric bacilli and enterococci may grow, but the colonies are usually small and translucent. Sucrose-fermenting *Proteus* strains produce yellow colonies that are similar to *Vibrio* colonies.

Tinsdale Agar

Tinsdale agar is a selective differential medium used for the isolation of *Corynebacterium diphtheriae* from upper respiratory specimens. The medium consists of peptones, salt, yeast extract, L-cysteine, potassium tellurite, and serum. The potassium tellurite inhibits the growth of most commensal organisms in the upper respiratory tract and allows the growth of *C. diphtheriae* and related *Corynebacterium* species. *C. diphtheriae* colonies can be distinguished by the brown halo that develops around the black colonies. These halos result from the reaction of tellurite with hydrogen sulfide, which *C. diphtheriae* produces from the cysteine in the medium.

Xylose-Lysine-Deoxycholate (XLD) Agar

Xylose-lysine-deoxycholate agar is a moderately selective medium used for the isolation and differentiation of enteric pathogens. The medium consists of yeast extract with xylose, lysine, lactose, sucrose, sodium deoxycholate, sodium thiosulfate, ferric ammonium citrate, and phenol red. The majority of the nonpathogenic enteric bacilli ferment lactose, sucrose, or xylose, producing yellow colonies (the phenol red indicator is yellow at acidic pH). Because *Shigella* spp. do not ferment these carbohydrates, the colonies are red. *Salmonella* and *Edwardsiella* spp. ferment xylose, but they also decarboxylate lysine to an alkaline diamine, cadaverine. This diamine neutralizes the acid products of fermentation by decarboxylation of lysine and produces red colonies. If the organism produces hydrogen sulfide (e.g., *Salmonella* and *Edwardsiella* spp.), the center of the colonies will blacken. Sodium deoxycholate inhibits the growth of many nonpathogenic organisms (in the presence of acid, it precipitates, producing yellow, opaque colonies).

Specimen Processing

Primary Plating Media: Mycobacteria

American Thoracic Society Medium

American Thoracic Society medium contains coagulated egg yolks, potato flour, glycerol, and malachite green. The concentration of malachite green is lower than in Lowenstein-Jensen (LJ) medium, allowing earlier detection of mycobacterial colonies, but the medium is also more easily overgrown by contaminants.

BACTEC 12B Broth

BACTEC 12B broth is used in the BACTEC AFB automated culture system. The formulation is Middlebrook 7H9 broth supplemented with albumin, casein hydrolysate, catalase, and ^{14}C-labeled palmitic acid. As the mycobacteria grow, palmitic acid is metabolized and $^{14}CO_2$ is released, which is detected by the BACTEC instrument. Contaminating bacteria are suppressed by the addition of polymyxin B, nalidixic acid, trimethoprim, azlocillin, and polyoxylene stearate.

BACTEC 13A Broth

BACTEC 13A broth medium is also used in the BACTEC system. The formulation is Middlebrook 7H12 medium supplemented with sodium polyanetholesulfonate. This broth can be used for blood and bone marrow aspirate specimens.

Dubos Broth

Dubos broth, a nonselective broth, contains casein digests, salt solutions, L-asparagine, ferric ammonium citrate, albumin or serum, and Tween 80. The growth of most species of mycobacteria is rapid in this medium, although the addition of antibiotics is required when specimens from contaminated sites are processed. Tween 80 is a surfactant that facilitates the dispersal of clumps of mycobacteria and results in more rapid, homogeneous growth.

Lowenstein-Jensen (LJ) Medium

Lowenstein-Jensen medium consists of glycerol, potato flour, defined salts, and coagulated whole eggs (to solidify the medium). Malachite green is added to inhibit contaminating bacteria, particularly gram-positive bacteria. LJ medium has a long shelf life (several months) and supports the growth of most mycobacteria, in part because lecithin in the eggs neutralizes many toxic factors present in clinical specimens. A problem with LJ medium is that the contaminants that grow on this medium can completely hydrolyze it.

Lowenstein-Jensen Medium, Gruft Modification
The Gruft modification of LJ medium contains RNA, penicillin, and nalidixic acid, which further suppress the growth of contaminating organisms. Because the growth of mycobacteria can be delayed with this selective medium, it should always be used with a tube of nonselective medium.

Lowenstein-Jensen Medium, Mycobactosel Modification
The Mycobactosel modification of LJ medium contains cycloheximide, lincomycin, and nalidixic acid to suppress the growth of contaminants.

Middlebrook 7H9 Broth
The 7H9 formulation of Middlebrook broth is the same as Middlebrook 7H10 agar, except that the agar and malachite green are absent. The growth of most mycobacteria is rapid in this medium, although antibiotics must be added to suppress the growth of contaminants.

Middlebrook 7H10 Agar
Middlebrook 7H10 agar is a nonselective medium that contains defined salts, vitamins, cofactors, oleic acid, albumin, catalase, glycerol, glucose, and malachite green. The addition of glycerol enhances the growth of *Mycobacterium avium-intracellulare*. Pyruvic acid can be added if *Mycobacterium bovis* is suspected, and 0.25% L-asparagine or 0.1% potassium aspartate must be added for maximal production of niacin. The medium has a relatively short shelf life (approximately 1 month), and exposure to heat or light may result in its deterioration and in release of formaldehyde. Growth of mycobacteria can be detected earlier on this medium than on egg-based media.

Middlebrook 7H10 Agar, Mycobactosel Modification
The Mycobactosel modification of Middlebrook 7H10 agar contains malachite green, cycloheximide, lincomycin, and nalidixic acid. As with the selective LJ media, the presence of antibiotics may delay the detection of mycobacteria, so a nonselective isolation medium should also be used.

Middlebrook 7H11 Agar

Middlebrook 7H11 agar is preferred over 7H10 agar because the addition of casein hydrolysates improves the recovery of isoniazid-resistant strains of *Mycobacterium tuberculosis*, which have become prevalent in some communities.

Middlebrook 7H11 Agar, Mitchison's Modification

Mitchison's modification of 7H11 medium contains carbenicillin, polymyxin B, trimethoprim, and amphotericin B. The carbenicillin is particularly useful for suppressing the growth of *Pseudomonas* spp.

Middlebrook 7H13 Broth

Middlebrook 7H13 broth is based on the 7H9 broth formulation supplemented with casein hydrolysate, polysorbate 80, sodium polyanetholesulfonate, catalase, and [^{14}C]palmitic acid. This broth is used in the BACTEC system.

Petragnani Medium

Petragnani medium is a nonselective mycobacterial medium that contains coagulated whole eggs, egg yolks, whole milk, potato, potato flour, glycerol, and malachite green. This medium is more inhibitory than LJ medium because it contains a higher concentration of malachite green. It should be restricted to use with heavily contaminated specimens.

Primary Plating Media: Fungi

Birdseed Agar

Birdseed (also called niger seed) agar is used for the selective isolation and identification of *Cryptococcus neoformans*. The agar medium contains an extract of *Guizotia abyssinica* seed, caffeic acid. *C. neoformans* produces phenol oxidase, and dark brown colonies develop in the presence of caffeic acid. The medium contains chloramphenicol to suppress the growth of bacteria.

Brain Heart Infusion Agar

Brain heart infusion agar is a nutritionally enriched medium that can be used for the isolation of a variety of fastidious bacteria, yeast, and molds. It is prepared with infusions of calf brains and beef hearts, peptones, glucose, sodium chloride, and disodium phosphate. Supplementation with 5 to 10% sheep blood can enrich the medium, and the addition of antibiotics (e.g., gentamicin, chloramphenicol, and penicillin) can make this medium selective for fungi.

CHROMagar *Candida*

CHROMagar *Candida* is a selective, differential agar medium for the isolation and presumptive identification of *Candida albicans*, *C. krusei*, and *C. tropicalis*. The medium consists of peptones, glucose, chloramphenicol, and "chromogenic mix." The antibiotic inhibits the growth of most bacteria. *C. albicans* forms green colonies, *C. krusei* forms pink colonies, and *C. tropicalis* forms purple colonies.

Dermatophyte Test Medium (DTM)

Dermatophyte test medium is a selective agar medium used for the isolation and identification of dermatophytes. It consists of digests of soybean meal supplemented with glucose, cycloheximide, chlortetracycline, gentamicin, and phenol red. The antibiotics suppress the growth of bacteria, saprophytic yeasts, and molds. Dermatophytes growing on this medium produce alkaline by-products that change the phenol red indicator from yellow to red. This color change may be obscured when grossly contaminated specimens (e.g., nails) are processed on this medium. The pigment produced by dermatophytes, which is used for their identification, is obscured by the intense red color produced on this medium.

Inhibitory Mold Agar (IMA)

Inhibitory mold agar is an enriched, selective medium that is used for the isolation of pathogenic fungi other than dermatophytes. It consists of digests of animal tissue and casein, yeast extract, dextrin, starch, glucose, salts, and chloramphenicol. Contaminating bacteria are inhibited by chloramphenicol.

Mycosel (Mycobiotic) Agar

Mycosel (Mycobiotic) agar is a selective medium used for the isolation of pathogenic fungi from contaminated specimens. Mycosel agar (BBL) and Mycobiotic agar (Difco) consist of digests of soybean meal supplemented with glucose, cycloheximide, and chloramphenicol. Cycloheximide-susceptible fungi, including *Cryptococcus neoformans*, *Pseudallescheria boydii*, the zygomycetes, many species of

Candida and *Aspergillus*, *Trichosporon beigelii*, and most saprophytic or opportunistic fungi, will not grow on this medium.

Sabouraud Agar-Brain Heart Infusion (SABHI)

Sabouraud agar-brain heart infusion (SABHI), an enriched agar medium, is a variation of Sabouraud dextrose agar (described below). The medium consists of infusions of beef heart and calf brains, peptones, salts, glucose, blood, and chloromycetin (chloramphenicol). It is used for the cultivation of dermatophytes and other pathogenic and nonpathogenic fungi.

Sabouraud Dextrose Agar (SDA)

Sabouraud dextrose agar is an enriched agar medium used for the isolation of saprophytic and pathogenic fungi. The original formulation of SDA consists of digests of casein and animal tissue supplemented with 4% glucose and adjusted to pH 5.6. The Emmons modification is preferred by many mycologists. It contains a reduced concentration of glucose (2%) and is buffered to neutrality (pH 6.9). Yeast, dermatophytes, and other filamentous fungi grow on these media. The original formulation of SDA was acidic to suppress the growth of bacteria. This problem can be circumvented by the addition of antibiotics (e.g., cycloheximide and chloramphenicol) to the media. However, cycloheximide-susceptible fungi (refer to Mycosel agar above) do not grow on this medium.

Yeast Extract-Phosphate Agar

Yeast extract-phosphate agar is a selective medium used for the isolation of pathogenic fungi such as *Histoplasma* and *Blastomyces* spp. It consists of yeast extract and phosphate buffer supplemented with chloramphenicol to suppress the growth of bacteria. The pH is adjusted to 6.0.

Table 4.1 Dyes and pH indicators

Indicator	pH and color	
Acid fuchsin (Andrade's)	5.0, pink	8.0, pale yellow
Bromcresol green	3.8, yellow	5.4, blue
Bromcresol purple	5.2, yellow	6.8, purple
Bromphenol blue	3.0, yellow	4.6, blue
Bromthymol blue	6.0, yellow	7.6, dark blue
Chlorcresol green	4.0, yellow	5.6, blue
Chlorphenol red	5.0, yellow	6.6, red
Cresolphthalein	8.2, colorless	9.8, red
m-Cresol purple	7.4, yellow	9.0, purple
Cresol red	7.2, yellow	8.8, red
Methyl red	4.4, red	6.2, yellow
Neutral red	6.8, red	8.0, yellow
Phenolphthalein	8.3, colorless	10.0, red
Phenol red	6.8, yellow	8.4, red
Thymol blue	8.0, yellow	9.6, blue
Resazurin	Oxidized: blue, nonfluorescent	Reduced: red, fluorescent
Triphenyl-tetrazolium chloride	Oxidized: colorless	Reduced: red

Specimen Processing

Table 4.2 Cells used for virus or *Chlamydia* isolation

Type of cell	Species or tissue of origin	Virus[b] or *Chlamydia* sp. isolated
Primary cells		
African green monkey	Kidney	HSV, mumps virus, RSV, rubella virus, VZV
CBMC, PBMC[a]	Human	HIV-1, HIV-2, HTLV-1, HTLV-2, HHV-6
Embryo fibroblasts	Chicken	Newcastle disease virus, human poxviruses
Embryonic kidney or lung	Human	Adenovirus, human polyomavirus BK, mumps virus, VZV
Rabbit	Kidney	HSV
Rhesus or cynomolgus monkey	Kidney	Echovirus, poliovirus, coxsackievirus groups A and B, mumps virus, reovirus, influenza virus, measles virus, parainfluenza virus, RSV
Finite cell lines		
Foreskin fibroblasts	Human	CMV, HSV
Kidney fibroblasts	Human, fetal	Coronavirus, HSV, rhinovirus
Lung fibroblasts	Human, embryo	Coronavirus, CMV, rhinovirus, VZV
WI-38, MRC-5	Human, fetal lung	Adenovirus, CMV, poliovirus, coxsackievirus group B, enterovirus (type 68-71), RSV, rhinovirus, HSV
Continuous cell lines		
293	Human kidney	Adenovirus (types 5, 40, 41)
A549	Human lung	Adenovirus (types 1 to 39)

(continued)

Specimen Processing

Table 4.2 Cells used for virus or *Chlamydia* isolation (*continued*)

Type of cell	Species or tissue of origin	Virus[b] or *Chlamydia* sp. isolated
BGMK	Buffalo green monkey kidney	Poliovirus, coxsackievirus groups A and B, reovirus, *C. trachomatis*
HeLa	Human cervix	*C. trachomatis*, poliovirus, poxvirus, reovirus, RSV, rhinovirus, coxsackievirus groups A and B
HEp-2	Human larynx	Adenovirus, RSV, *C. pneumoniae*
McCoy	Mouse	*C. trachomatis*, *C. psittaci*
MDCK	Canine kidney	Influenza virus, parainfluenza virus
Mink lung	Mink	HSV
Rhabdomyosarcoma (RD)	Human	Coronavirus, coxsackievirus group A, poliovirus, enterovirus (types 68 to 71)
RK_{13}	Rabbit kidney	Rubella virus, poxvirus
Vero, CV-1	African green monkey kidney	HSV, measles virus, poxvirus, human polyomavirus BK, rubella virus, RSV, parainfluenza virus

[a]CBMC, cord blood mononuclear cells; PBMC, peripheral blood mononuclear cells.
[b]CMV, cytomegalovirus; HSV, herpes simplex virus; HHV-6, human herpesvirus 6; HIV-1 and -2, human immunodeficiency virus types 1 and 2; HTLV-1 and -2, human T-lymphotropic virus types 1 and 2; RSV, respiratory syncytial virus; VZV, varicella-zoster virus.

Microscopy

Acid-Fast Trichrome Chromotrope Stain

The acid-fast trichrome chromotrope stain is used to detect microsporidia and *Cryptosporidium* and *Isospora* spp. Specimens are stained first with carbol fuchsin and then with Didier's trichrome solution (Chromotrope 2R, aniline blue, and phosphotungstic acid in acetic acid) and then washed with acid-alcohol followed by 95% ethanol. Oocysts of *Cryptosporidium* and *Isospora* spp. stain bright pink or violet, and microsporidia appear pink.

Acridine Orange Stain

Acridine orange is a fluorescent dye that intercalates into nucleic acid (native and the denatured). At neutral pH, bacteria, fungi, and cellular material (e.g., leukocytes, squamous epithelial cells) stain red-orange. At acidic pH (pH 4.0), bacteria and fungi remain red-orange, but the background material stains green-yellow. Optimal detection of fluorescence requires the use of a 420- to 490-nm excitation filter and a 520-nm barrier filter.

Auramine-Rhodamine Stain

Auramine and rhodamine are fluorochromes that bind to mycolic acids and are resistant to decolorization with acid alcohol (acid-fast stain). Acid-fast organisms appear orange-yellow. Potassium permanganate is used as a counterstain. It is a strong oxidizing agent that inactivates the unbound fluorochrome dyes, producing a black background for the stained specimens. Fluorochrome-stained smears can be restained by the Kinyoun or Ziehl-Neelsen methods. Optimal detection of fluorescence requires use of a 420- to 490-nm excitation filter and a 520-nm barrier filter.

Calcofluor White Stain

Calcofluor white is a nonspecific fluorochrome that binds to cellulose and chitin in the cell walls of fungi. The dye can be mixed with 10% potassium hydroxide so that mammalian cells can be dissolved, thus facilitating visualization of fungal elements. Fungi, *Pneumocystis carinii*, and *Acanthamoeba* spp. will appear green or blue against a dark background when the stained slide is examined under UV illumination. Care must be used to distinguish specific staining from stained debris. Optimal detection of fluorescence requires the use of a 400- to 500-nm excitation filter and 500- to 520-nm barrier filter.

Direct Fluorescent-Antibody Stain

A variety of organisms (e.g., *Streptococcus pyogenes*, *Bordetella pertussis*, *Francisella tularensis*, *Legionella* spp., *Chlamydia trachomatis*, *Cryptosporidium parvum*, *Giardia lamblia*, influenza virus, and herpes simplex virus) are directly detected in clinical specimens by using specific fluorescein-labeled antibodies. The labeled antibodies bind to the organisms and fluoresce green under UV light. The sensitivity and specificity of the stain are determined by the quality of the antibodies used in the reagents. Optimal detection of fluorescence requires the use of either a 420- to 490-nm (wide-band) or 470- to 490-nm (narrow-band) excitation filter and a 510- to 530-nm barrier filter.

Giemsa Stain

Giemsa stain, like Wright stain, is a modification of Romanowsky stain, which combines methylene blue and eosin. Both stains are used for the detection of blood parasites (e.g., *Plasmodium*, *Babesia*, and *Leishmania* spp.), fungi (e.g., *Histoplasma* yeast cells and *Pneumocystis carinii*), rickettsiae, chlamydiae, and viral inclusions. A protozoan trophozoite has a red nucleus and gray-blue cytoplasm; intracellular yeasts and inclusions typically stain blue (basophilic), and rickettsiae, *Chlamydia* elementary bodies, and *P. carinii* stain purple.

Gram Stain

Gram stain is the most commonly used stain in clinical microbiology laboratories. It is used to separate bacteria into gram-positive (blue) and gram-negative (red) groups, as well as to detect fungi and many parasites. Variations in the performance of this stain are commonplace; however, the staining principle is constant. After the specimen is fixed to a glass slide (by either heating or treatment with 95% methanol), it is exposed to the basic dye crystal violet. Iodine is added and forms a complex with the primary dye. During the decolorization step, this complex is retained in gram-positive organisms but lost in gram-negative organisms. The gram-negative organisms are detected with a counterstain (e.g., safranin). The degree to which an organism retains the stain is a function of the species, culture conditions, and staining skills of the microbiologist. Older cultures tend to decolorize readily.

India Ink Stain (Nigrosin)

The use of India ink is not technically a staining method. Detection of encapsulated fungi (i.e., *Cryptococcus neoformans*) is made possible by exclusion of the ink particles by the polysaccharide capsule of the organism. Care in interpretation is required because artifacts (e.g., leukocytes, erythrocytes, powder, and bubbles) may be confused with yeast cells. The morphologic characteristics of the yeast cells must be recognized before the preparation can be interpreted.

Iron Hematoxylin Stain

Iron hematoxylin stain is used for the detection and identification of fecal protozoa. Helminth eggs and larvae generally retain too much stain and are more easily identified with wet-mount preparations. Iron hematoxylin stain can be applied to either fresh stool specimens or ones preserved with polyvinyl alcohol or a similar preservative. Formalin-fixed specimens cannot be used.

Kinyoun Stain

The presence of long-chain fatty acids (e.g., mycolic acid) in some organisms makes these organisms both difficult to stain with water-soluble dyes and resistant to decolorization with acid solutions (acid-fast). The Kinyoun method of staining uses phenol to facilitate the penetration of basic carbol fuchsin into the cells. This stain is also referred to as a cold acid-fast stain because the specimen does not have to be heated for the stain to penetrate, as it does with the Ziehl-Neelsen stain. Basic carbol fuchsin is used as the primary stain, 3% sulfuric acid in 95% ethanol (acid-alcohol) is the decolorizing agent, and methylene blue is the counterstain. Acid-fast organisms appear pink-red on a pale blue background. The contrast between organisms and background is sometimes poor, and the fluorochrome stain is generally preferred for specimen examination. Acid-fast stains are used for detecting bacteria including *Mycobacterium*, *Nocardia*, *Rhodococcus*, *Tsukamurella*, and *Gordona* spp. and the oocysts of *Cryptosporidium*, *Isopora*, *Sarcocystis*, and *Cyclospora* spp. Because some of these organisms lose the primary stain when exposed to 3% sulfuric acid, the decolorizing agent can be reduced to 0.5 to 1%. Organisms that retain this modified stain are referred to as being partially acid-fast.

Lugol's Iodine Stain
Iodine is added to "wet" preparations of parasitology specimens to enhance the contrast of the internal structures (e.g., nuclei and glycogen vacuoles). One disadvantage of this method is that protozoa are killed by the iodine and hence motility cannot be observed.

Methenamine Silver Stain
Methenamine silver staining is generally performed in surgical pathology laboratories rather than microbiology laboratories. It is used primarily for the detection of fungal elements in tissues, although other organisms (e.g., *Legionella* spp.) can be detected. Silver staining requires skill, because nonspecific staining can render the slide uninterpretable.

Methylene Blue Stain
Methylene blue is another contrasting dye commonly used in the laboratory, primarily for the detection of bacteria and fungi. It can be mixed with potassium hydroxide and used to examine skin scrapings for fungal elements.

Periodic Acid-Schiff (PAS) Stain
Periodic acid-Schiff stain is used to detect yeast cells and fungal hyphae in tissues. Periodic acid (5%) hydrolyzes the cell wall aldehydes, which then combine with the modified Schiff reagent and stain the cell wall carbohydrates pink-magenta against a light green background. Because this staining procedure is complex, most laboratories use calcofluor white stain instead.

Potassium Hydroxide (KOH)
A 10 to 15% solution of potassium hydroxide can be used to dissolve cellular and organic debris and facilitate the detection of fungal elements, which are not affected by strong alkali solutions (although fungal elements dissolve after exposure for a few days). Ink (e.g., permanent blue-black Parker Super Quick Ink) can be added as a contrasting agent to aid the detection of fungi. Lactophenol cotton blue (i.e., Poirrier's blue) can also be added to the KOH. The aniline blue stains the outer cell wall of fungi, and the lactic acid is a clearing agent.

Toluidine Blue-O Stain

Toluidine blue-O stain is used primarily for the detection of *Pneumocystis carinii* in respiratory specimens. *P. carinii* cysts stain reddish blue to dark purple against a light blue background. Trophozoites do not stain by this method. This staining method is rapid and inexpensive, but some skill is required to recognize *P. carinii* cysts (usually present in clumps). Many laboratories prefer the direct fluorescent-antibody test for the detection of *P. carinii* even though the stain is more expensive.

Trichrome Stain

Trichrome stain, like the iron hematoxylin stain, is used for the detection and identification of protozoa. The stain consists of a solution of three dyes (Chromotrope 2R, light green SF, and fast green FCF) in phosphotungstic acid and acetic acid. When staining is done properly, the specimen background is green and the protozoa have a blue-green to purple cytoplasm with red or purple-red nuclei, chromatoid bodies, erythrocytes, and bacteria. Parasite eggs and larvae usually stain red.

Wright Stain

Wright stain is a polychromatic stain that contains a mixture of methylene blue, azure B (from the oxidation of methylene blue), and eosin Y dissolved in methanol. The eosin ions are negatively charged and stain the basic components of cells orange to pink, while the other dyes stain the acidic cell structures various shades of blue to purple.

Ziehl-Neelsen Stain

Ziehl-Neelsen stain is an acid-fast stain which requires that the specimen be heated during staining so that the basic carbol fuchsin can penetrate into the organisms. Once this penetration is accomplished, decolorization and counterstaining are the same as for the Kinyoun method. The sensitivity and specificity of this stain are essentially the same as those of the Kinyoun method.

Specimen Processing

Table 4.3 Recommendations for primary stains and bacterial culture media

	Stain[a]		Culture medium[b]													
Type of specimen	Gram	AFB	BA	CHOC	MAC, EMB	TM, NYC	BLD-B	A-BA	BBE	LKV	A-CNA, A-PEA	THIO, CMB	XLD, HE	CAMPY	CIN	S-MAC
Abscess	R	O	×	×	×			×	×	×	×					
Catheter	N	N	×	×												
Ear																
External	O	N	×	×	×											
Internal	R	N	×	×	×											
Eye																
External	O	N	×	×												
Internal	R	N	×	×												
Fluids																
Amniotic	R	O	×	×	×		×	×	×	×	×					
Blood	N	N					×									
Bone marrow	R	O	×	×			×									
Cerebrospinal	R	O	×	×								×				
Culdocentesis	R	O	×	×	×		×	×	×	×	×					
Paracentesis (abdominal)	R	O	×	×	×		×	×	×	×	×					
Pericardial	R	O	×	×			×									
Pleural	R	O	×	×			×	×				×				
Synovial (joint)	R	O	×	×			×					×				
Thoracentesis (chest)	R	O	×	×	×		×	×			×					

Source													
Gastrointestinal													
Bile	O	N	×	×							×		×	×
Colostomy	O	N	×	×							×		×	×
Gastric washing	O	N	×	×					×					
Ileostomy	O	N	×	×							×	×	×	×
Rectal swab	O	N	×	×							×	×	×	×
Stool (feces)	O	N	×	×							×	×	×	
Genital														
Cervix	O	N	×	×	×									
Prostate	R	O	×	×	×									
Urethra	O	N	×	×	×									
Uterus	O	N	×	×	×		×							
Vagina	O	N	×	×	×									
Respiratory														
Bronchial (brush, wash, lavage)	R	O	×	×	×									
Lung	R	O	×	×	×	×	×	×						
Mouth	O	N	×	×	×									
Nasal sinuses	R	N	×	×	×	×	×							
Nasopharynx	O	N	×	×	×									
Sputum	R	O	×	×	×									
Tracheal suction	R	O	×	×	×	×								
Transtracheal aspirate	R	O	×	×	×	×								

(continued)

Specimen Processing

Table 4.3 Recommendations for primary stains and bacterial culture media *(continued)*

Type of specimen	Stain[a] Gram	Stain[a] AFB	BA	CHOC	MAC, EMB	TM, NYC	BLD-B	A-BA	BBE	LKV	A-CNA, A-PEA	THIO, CMB	XLD, HE	CAMPY	CIN	S-MAC
Skin																
Superficial (e.g., cellulitis)	O	O	×	×	×											
Other (sinus tract, ulcer, fistula)	O	O	×	×	×											
Tissue																
Autopsy	O	O	×	×	×											
Burn	O	O	×	×	×											
Surgical	R	O	×	×	×			×	×	×	×	×				
Other (e.g., biopsy)	O	O	×	×	×			×	×	×	×	×				
Urine																
Catheterized	O	O	×		×											
Midstream voided	O	O	×		×											
Suprapubic aspirate	R	O	×		×		×									

[a] AFB, acid-fast bacillus; R, staining should be routinely performed; O, staining is optional and should be performed if requested; N, staining should not be performed unless the request is discussed with the physician.

[b] Abbreviations: BA, aerobic blood agar; CHOC, chocolate agar; MAC, MacConkey agar; EMB, eosin-methylene blue agar (either can be used); TM, NYC, Thayer-Martin agar and New York City agar (either can be used); BLD-B, blood culture bottle (used if more than 3 to 4 ml of fluid is received for processing); A-BA, anaerobic blood agar; BBE, *Bacteroides* bile esculin agar; LKV, kanamycin-vancomycin laked blood agar; A-CNA, A-PEA, anaerobic colistin-nalidixic agar and anaerobic phenylethyl alcohol agar (either can be used); THIO, CMB, thioglycolate broth and chopped-meat broth (either can be used); XLD, HE, xylose-lysine-deoxycholate agar and Hektoen enteric agar (either can be used); CAMPY, *Campylobacter* agar; CIN, cefsulodin-Irgasan-novobiocin agar; S-MAC, sorbitol-MacConkey agar.

Table 4.4 Recommendations for primary stains and fungal culture media

Type of specimen	Stain[a]		Culture medium[b]				
	KOH, CW	II	BHIA	BHIA-A, MYCO	IMA	BHIB	DTM
Abscess	R	N		X	X		
Catheter	N	N		X	X		
Ear	O	N		X	X		
Eye							
Corneal scraping	R	N		X		X	
Aspirate	R	N	X			X	
Fluids							
Blood	N	N	X				
Bone marrow	R	N	X		X		
Cerebrospinal	N	R	X			X	
Paracentesis	O	N	X		X		
Pleural	O	N	X		X		
Synovial	O	N	X		X		
Thoracentesis	O	N	X		X		

(continued)

Specimen Processing

Table 4.4 Recommendations for primary stains and fungal culture media (*continued*)

Type of specimen	Stain[a]		Culture medium[b]				
	KOH, CW	II	BHIA	BHIA-A, MYCO	IMA	BHIB	DTM
Gastrointestinal							
Gastric washing	N	N		X	X		
Rectal swab	N	N		X	X		
Stool (feces)	N	N		X	X		
Genital							
Cervix	O	N		X	X		
Vagina	O	N		X	X		
Respiratory							
Bronchial (brush, wash, lavage)	O	O		X	X		
Lung	O	O		X	X		
Mouth	O	N		X	X		
Nasal sinuses	O	N		X	X	X	
Nasopharynx	O	N		X	X		
Sputum	O	O		X	X		

Specimen						
Tracheal suction	O	O	X	X		
Transtracheal aspirate	O	O	X	X		
Skin						
Hair	R	N	X	X	X	X
Nails	R	N	X	X	X	X
Skin scrapings	R	N	X	X	X	X
Tissue						
Autopsy	O	N	X	X		
Burn	O	N	X	X		
Surgical	O	O	X	X		
Urine	O	O	X	X		

[a]KOH, 10 to 15% potassium hydroxide with Parker Super Quick permanent black ink; CW, calcofluor white; II, India ink; R, staining should be routinely performed; O, staining is optional and should be performed if requested; N, staining should not be performed unless the request is discussed with the physician.

[b]BHIA, brain heart infusion agar with blood; BHIA-A, MYCO, brain heart infusion agar supplemented with blood, gentamicin, chloramphenicol, and cycloheximide, and Mycosel or Mycobiotic agar (Sabourand dextrose agar with cycloheximide and chloramphenicol) (one or more of these selective media can be used); IMA, inhibitory mold agar (with chloramphenicol); BHIB, brain heart infusion broth; DTM, dermatophyte test medium.

Specimen Processing

Table 4.5 Selection of diagnostic tests for specific viral diseases

Disease and virus	Diagnostic tests[a]			
	Microscopy	Culture	Antigen tests	Antibody tests
Mycocarditis				
Adenoviruses	+	+	±	±
Arenaviruses	0	0	0	+
Enteroviruses	0	+	±	±
Flaviviruses	0	0	0	+
Herpesviruses	+	+	+	±
Influenza viruses	+	+	±	+
Measles virus	±	±	+	+
Mumps virus	0		+	+
Pericarditis				
Adenoviruses	+	+	±	±
Coxsackieviruses	0	+	±	±
Echoviruses	0	+	±	±
Herpesviruses	+	+	+	±
Influenza viruses	+	+	+	+
Mumps virus	0	±	+	+

Transfusion sepsis

Colorado tick fever virus	0	0	0	+
Cytomegalovirus	+	+	+	+
Epstein-Barr virus	±	±	+	+
Hepatitis viruses (A, B, C, D)	0	0	+	+
Human immunodeficiency virus	0	±	+	+
Parvovirus B19	±	0	+	+

Encephalitis

Adenoviruses	+	+	±	±
Alphaviruses	0	0	0	+
Arenaviruses	0	0	0	+
Bunyaviruses	0	0	0	+
Enteroviruses	0	+	±	±
Filoviruses	0	0	0	+
Flaviviruses	0	0	0	+
Herpesviruses	+	+	+	±
Human immunodeficiency virus	0	±	±	+
Measles virus	±	+	+	+
Mumps virus	0	±	+	+
Rabies virus	±	0	0	+
Rubella virus	0	±	+	+

(continued)

Specimen Processing

Table 4.5 Selection of diagnostic tests for specific viral diseases *(continued)*

Disease and virus	Diagnostic tests[a]			
	Microscopy	Culture	Antigen tests	Antibody tests
Meningitis				
Colorado tick fever virus	0	0	0	+
Enteroviruses	0	+	±	±
Flaviviruses	0	0	0	+
Herpes simplex virus	+	+	+	±
Human immunodeficiency virus	0	±	+	+
Lymphocytic choriomeningitis virus	0	0	0	+
Mumps virus	0	±	+	+
Otitis media				
Enteroviruses	0	+	±	±
Influenza viruses	+	+	+	+
Respiratory syncytial virus	+	+	+	+
Rhinoviruses	0	+	±	0
Conjunctivitis				
Adenoviruses	+	+	±	±
Enteroviruses	0	+	±	±
Herpesviruses	+	+	+	±
Influenza viruses	+	+	+	+

Measles virus	±	+	±	+
Papillomaviruses	±	0	+	0
Rubella virus	0	±	+	+
Keratitis				
Adenoviruses	+	+	±	±
Herpesviruses	+	+	+	±
Measles virus	±	+	±	+
Endophthalmitis				
Herpesviruses	+	+	+	±
Measles virus	±	+	±	+
Rubella virus	0	±	+	+
Sinusitis				
Adenoviruses	+	+	±	±
Influenza viruses	+	+	+	+
Parainfluenza viruses	+	+	+	±
Rhinoviruses	0	+	±	0
Pharyngitis				
Adenoviruses	+	+	±	±
Coxsackieviruses	0	+	±	±
Herpesviruses	+	+	+	±
Human immunodeficiency virus	0	±	+	+

(continued)

Specimen Processing

Specimen Processing

Table 4.5 Selection of diagnostic tests for specific viral diseases *(continued)*

Disease and virus	Diagnostic tests[a]			
	Microscopy	Culture	Antigen tests	Antibody tests
Influenza viruses	+	+	+	+
Parainfluenza viruses	+	+	+	+|
Respiratory syncytial virus	+	+	+	+
Rhinoviruses	0	+	+|	0
Laryngotracheobronchitis				
Influenza viruses	+	+	+	+
Parainfluenza viruses	+	+	+	+|
Respiratory syncytial virus	+	+	+	+
Bronchitis				
Adenoviruses	+	+	+|	+|
Coxsackievirus type A	0	+|	+|	+|
Influenza viruses	+	+	+	+
Parainfluenza viruses	+	+	+	+|
Respiratory syncytial virus	+	+	+	+
Rhinoviruses	0	+	+|	0
Pneumonia				
Adenoviruses	+	+	+|	+|
Enteroviruses	0	+	+|	+|

Herpesviruses	+	+	+	+	±
Influenza viruses	+	+	+	+	+
Measles virus	±	+	±	+	+
Parainfluenza viruses	+	+	+	+	±
Respiratory syncytial virus	+	+	+	+	+
Rhinoviruses	0	0	+	±	0
Gastrointestinal infections					
Adenoviruses	0	+	+	0	±
Astroviruses	+	0	0	+	0
Caliciviruses	+	0	0	+	0
Coronaviruses	+	0	0	+	0
Cytomegalovirus	+	+	+	+	+
Rotaviruses	+	0	0	+	0
Genitourinary infections					
Adenoviruses	0	±	±	+	±
Cytomegalovirus	+	+	+	+	+
Herpes simplex virus	+	+	+	+	±
Measles virus	±	0	±	+	0
Papillomaviruses	±	0	+	0	0
Maculopapular rash					
Alphaviruses	0	0	0	0	+

(continued)

Specimen Processing

Table 4.5 Selection of diagnostic tests for specific viral diseases *(continued)*

Disease and virus	Diagnostic tests[a]			
	Microscopy	Culture	Antigen tests	Antibody tests
Bunyaviruses	0	0	0	+
Enteroviruses	0	+	±	±
Flaviviruses	0	0	0	+
Hepatitis B virus	0	0	+	+
Herpesviruses	+	+	+	±
Measles virus	±	+	±	+
Rubella virus	0	±	+	+
Parvovirus B19	±	0	+	+
Vesicular rash				
Enteroviruses	0	+	±	±
Herpes simplex virus	+	+	+	±
Varicella-zoster virus	+	+	+	+
Nodular rash				
Papillomaviruses	±	0	+	0
Molluscum contagiosum virus	0	0	±	0
Orf virus	0	0	±	0

[a]Diagnostic tests: +, primary diagnostic test; ±, secondary test; 0, not useful.

Table 4.6 Selection of diagnostic tests for specific parasitic diseases

Body site and parasite	Microscopy						Culture	Antigen test[b]	Antibody test
	Wet mount	Permanent stain[a]	Acid-fast stain	Calcofluor stain	Giemsa stain	DFA stain			
Blood/bone marrow									
Babesia spp.					×				
Leishmania spp.					×		×	×	
Microfilariae		×			×			×	
Plasmodium spp.					×		×	×	
Toxoplasma gondii					×		×	×	×
Trypanosoma cruzi					×		×	×	×
Eyes									
Acanthamoeba spp.	×	×		×			×	×	
Loa loa					×				
Microsporidia		×	×	×	×			×	
Toxoplasma gondii					×		×	×	×
Central nervous system									
Acanthamoeba spp.	×	×		×			×	×	
Balamuthia spp.	×	×					×	×	

(continued)

Specimen Processing

Table 4.6 Selection of diagnostic tests for specific parasitic diseases (continued)

Body site and parasite	Microscopy						Culture	Antigen test[b]	Antibody test
	Wet mount	Permanent stain[a]	Acid-fast stain	Calcofluor stain	Giemsa stain	DFA stain			
Echinococcus spp.	X								X
Microsporidia		X	X	X				X	
Naegleria fowleri	X	X	X	X			X		
Plasmodium falciparum					X			X	X
Taenia solium	X								X
Toxoplasma gondii					X		X	X	X
Trypanosoma spp.					X		X	X	X
Liver and spleen									
Echinococcus spp.	X							X	X
Entamoeba histolytica	X	X					X	X	X
Leishmania spp.					X		X	X	
Microsporidia		X	X	X	X			X	
Muscle									
Microsporidia			X	X	X			X	
Onchocerca volvulus	X								
Taenia solium	X								X

Trichinella spiralis			×			×	×
Trypanosoma cruzi			×	×	×	×	×
Intestinal tract							
Balantidium coli	×						
Cestodes	×						
Cryptosporidium spp.	×			×		×	
Cyclospora spp.	×				×	×	
Entamoeba spp.	×					×	×
Giardia lamblia	×			×	×	×	
Isospora belli	×						
Microsporidia	×	×	×			×	
Nematodes	×						
Trematodes	×						
Lungs							
Ascaris lumbricoides	×					×	
Cryptosporidium spp.	×			×		×	
Echinococcus spp.	×						
Entamoeba histolytica	×	×	×			×	
Microsporidia					×	×	×
Paragonimus spp.	×						×

(continued)

Table 4.6 Selection of diagnostic tests for specific parasitic diseases (*continued*)

Body site and parasite	Microscopy						Culture	Antigen test[b]	Antibody test
	Wet mount	Permanent stain[a]	Acid-fast stain	Calcofluor stain	Giemsa stain	DFA stain			
Strongyloides spp.	×								
Toxoplasma gondii					×		×	×	×
Skin/cutaneous ulcers									
Acanthamoeba spp.	×	×		×			×	×	
Entamoeba histolytica	×	×					×	×	×
Leishmania spp.					×		×	×	
Mansonella spp.	×	×					×	×	
Microfilaria		×		×	×			×	
Onchocerca volvulus	×								
Urogenital system									
Enterobius spp.	×	×							
Microsporidia		×	×	×	×			×	
Schistosoma spp.	×								
Trichomonas vaginalis	×				×		×	×	

[a]Permanent stains: trichrome, modified trichrome, and iron hematoxylin.
[b]Antigen tests: immunoassays and PCR-based tests.

Specimen Processing

Microbial Identification

A major function of clinical microbiology laboratories is microbial identification. The identity of an organism can be used to assess its clinical significance, the epidemiology of an infection, and the selection of empiric therapy. Frequently, significant delays occur before the definitive identification is obtained. Therefore, knowledge of the characteristic morphologic and physiologic properties of the most likely organisms to be associated with specific diseases can be used to provide a rapid, preliminary identification of an isolate. This, in turn, can be used to guide the empiric treatment of a patient.

The extensive list of microbes that can colonize humans or cause human disease makes it difficult to provide a comprehensive identification scheme in this guidebook. However, rules for the identification of the most common bacteria, fungi, and parasites are presented in this section. Virus identification is not discussed here because viruses are identified by their growth in specific eukaryotic cells (refer to section 4) and immunologic testing (refer to section 7). For a definitive approach to organism identification, the reader is referred to the references listed in the Bibliography. A particularly useful resource is the *Manual of Clinical Microbiology*.

The following symbols are used throughout this section. Test reactivity: 0, <10% of the tests are positive; +, >90% of the tests are positive; V, test reactions are variable; NT, organism was not tested in the specific reaction; S, organism is susceptible to the antibiotic or reagent; R, organism is resistant to the antibiotic or reagent. Metabolic products (GLC): A, acetic acid; P, propionic acid; IB, isobutyric acid; B, butyric acid; IV, isovaleric acid; V, valeric acid; IC, isocaproic acid; C, caproic acid; L, lactic acid; S, succinic acid. Capital letters indicate a major acid peak, lowercase letters indicate a minor peak, and letters in parentheses indicate that the acids are irregularly observed.

Microbial Identification

Table 5.1 Differential characteristics of catalase-positive, gram-positive cocci

Genus	Vancomycin susceptibility	Atmosphere[a]	Growth in 5% NaCl	Oxidase	Cell type[b]
Staphylococcus	S	F	+	−	cl, pr
Stomatococcus[c]	S	F	−	−	cl, pr
Micrococcus	S	Ae	+	+	cl, te
Alloiococcus	S	Ae	+	−	cb, pr, te

[a]F, facultative anaerobe; Ae, aerobe.
[b]cb, coccobacilli; cl, clusters; pr, pairs; te, tetrads.
[c]Genus with negative, weakly positive, and strongly positive catalase reactions.

Microbial Identification

Table 5.2 Differential characteristics of common *Staphylococcus* species

Staphylococcus species	Colony pigment	Coagulase	Clumping factor	Acid from: Cellobiose	Maltose	Mannitol	Mannose	Sucrose	Trehalose	Turanose	Xylose	Heat-stable nuclease	Alkaline phosphatase	PYR[a] hydrolysis	Ornithine decarboxylase	Urease	β-Galactosidase	Voges-Proskauer	Novobiocin	Polymyxin B
S. aureus	+	+	+	−	+	+	+	+	+	+	−	+	+	−	−	V	−	+	S	R
S. epidermidis	−	−	−	−	+	−	+	+	−	V	−	−	+	−	V	+	−	+	S	R
S. haemolyticus	V	−	−	−	+	V	−	+	+	V	−	−	−	+	−	−	−	+	S	S
S. hyicus	−	V	−	−	−	−	+	+	+	−	−	+	+	−	−	V	−	−	S	R
S. intermedius	−	+	V	−	V	V	+	+	+	V	−	+	+	+	−	+	+	−	S	S
S. lugdunensis	V	−	+	−	+	−	+	+	+	V	−	−	−	+	+	V	−	+	S	V
S. saprophyticus	V	−	−	−	+	V	−	+	+	+	−	−	−	−	−	+	+	+	R	S
S. schleiferi	−	−	+	−	−	−	+	−	V	−	−	+	+	+	−	−	+	+	S	S

[a]PYR, pyrrolidonyl arylamidase.

Table 5.3 Differential characteristics of catalase-negative, pyrrolidonyl arylamidase-negative, gram-positive cocci

Genus	Vancomycin susceptibility	Leucine aminopeptidase	Growth: 10°C	Growth: 45°C	Growth: 6.5% NaCl	cell types[a]
Leuconostoc	R	−	+	V	V	cb, pr, ch
Pediococcus	R	+	−	+	V	pr, cl, te
Lactococcus	S	+	+	−	V	ch, cb, pr
Streptococcus	S	+	−	V	−	ch, pr
Aerococcus[b]	S	+	−	−	+	te, pr, cl
Stomatococcus[c]	S	+	−	−	−	cl, pr

[a]cb, coccobacilli; ch, chains; cl, clusters; pr, pairs; te, tetrads.
[b]*Aerococcus urinae.*
[c]Pyrrolidonyl arylamidase (PYR)-negative strains are uncommon.

Microbial Identification

Microbial Identification

Table 5.4 Differential characteristics of catalase-negative, pyrrolidonyl arylamidase-positive, gram-positive cocci

Genus	Vancomycin susceptibility	Leucine aminopeptidase	Growth:				Bile-esculin	Cell types[a]
			6.5% NaCl	10°C	45°C			
Enterococcus	V	+	+	+	+	+	ch, pr
Lactococcus	S	+	V	+	–	+	ch, cb, pr
Stomatococcus[b]	S	+	–	–	–	–	cl, pr
Abiotrophia[c]	S	+	–	–	–	–	ch, pr
Gemella[d]	S	V	–	–	–	–	pr
Globicatella	S	–	+	–	–	–	cb, ch, pr
Helcococcus	S	–	+	–	–	+	pr, cl
Aerococcus[e]	S	–	+	–	+	V	te, pr, cl

[a]cb, coccobacilli; ch, chains; cl, clusters; pr, pairs; te, tetrads.
[b]Mucoid colonies adherent to agar surface.
[c]Nutritionally deficient colonies with satellite growth around staphylococci.
[d]Diplococci with flattened sides resembling *Neisseria* species.
[e]*Aerococcus viridans*; poor anaerobic growth.

Table 5.5 Differential characteristics of beta-hemolytic streptococci

Streptococcus species	Lancefield group	Pyrrolidonyl arylamidase (PYR)	Bacitracin	Voges-Proskauer	CAMP test	Hippurate	β-Glucuronidase
S. pyogenes	A	+	+	−	−	−	NT
S. agalactiae	B	−	−	−	+	+	NT
S. dysgalactiae subsp. *equisimilis*	C	−	−	−	−	−	+
S. anginosus group	A, B, C, F, G, nongrp	−	−	+	−	−	−

Microbial Identification

Table 5.6 Differential characteristics of selected viridans streptococci[a]

Streptococcus species	Acid from:						Hydrolysis of:		Voges-Proskauer
	Inulin	Mannitol	Raffinose	Sorbitol	Lactose	Melibiose	Arginine	Esculin	
S. sanguis	V	–	V	V	+	V	+	V	–
S. gordonii	+	–	–	–	+	–	+	+	+
S. oralis	–	–	V	–	+	V	–	V	–
S. mitis	–	–	+	–	V	+	–	–	–
S. anginosus group	–	–	–	–	V	V	+	V	+
S. mutans	+	+	+	+	+	+	–	V	+
S. sobrinus	–	+	–	V	+	–	–	–	+
S. salivarius	V	–	V	–	+	–	–	+	+
S. bovis	+	+	+	–	+	+	–	+	+

[a]*Streptococcus pneumoniae* resembles these bacteria and is identified by bile solubility and susceptibility to optochin.

Table 5.7 Differential characteristics of *Enterococcus* groups

Group	Acid from: Mannitol	Acid from: Sorbitol	Arginine dihydrolase
I	+	+	−
II	+	−	+
III	−	−	+
IV	−	−	−
V	+	−	−

Microbial Identification

Table 5.8 Differential characteristics of common *Enterococcus* species

Group	Species	Acid from: Arabinose	Sorbitol	Raffinose	Sucrose	Pyruvate	Growth in 0.04% tellurite	Motility	Pigment production	Methyl-α-D-glucopyranoside	Efrotomycin susceptibility (100 μg)
I	*E. avium*	+	+	−	+	+	−	−	−	+	R
	E. raffinosus	+	+	+	+	+	−	−	−	+	R
	E. pseudoavium	−	+	−	+	+	−	−	−	+	R
II	*E. faecalis*	−	>	>	+	+	+	−	−	−	R
	E. faecium	+	>	+	+	−	−	−	−	−	S
	E. casseliflavus	+	−	+	+	>	−	+	+	+	R
	E. gallinarum	+	−	+	−	−	−	+	−	+	R
III	*E. durans*	−	−	−	+	−	−	−	−	−	S
	E. hirae	−	−	>	+	−	−	−	−	−	S
	E. dispar	−	−	+	+	−	−	−	−	+	R
	E. faecalis variant	−	−	−	>	+	+	−	−	−	R
	E. faecium variant	+	−	>	+	+	−	−	−	−	S

Table 5.9 Differential characteristics of selected *Corynebacterium* species

Species	Nitrate reductase	Urease	Esculin hydrolysis	Pyrazinamidase	Alkaline phosphatase	Acid from: Glucose	Maltose	Sucrose	Mannitol	Xylose
Oxidative										
C. jeikeium[a]	–	–	–	+	+	+	v	–	–	–
C. urealyticum[a]	–	+	–	–	v	–	–	–	–	–
C. pseudodiphtheriticum	+	+	–	+	–	–	–	–	–	–
C. afermentans	–	–	–	+	+	–	–	–	–	–
C. mucifaciens	–	–	–	+	+	+	–	v	–	–
Fermentative										
C. diphtheriae	+	–	–	–	–	+	+	–	–	–
C. ulcerans	–	+	–	–	–	+	+	–	–	–
C. amycolatum[a]	v	v	–	+	+	+	v	v	–	–
C. coyleae	–	–	–	+	+	+	–	–	–	–
C. macginleyi[a]	+	–	–	–	+	+	–	+	–	–
C. minutissimum	–	–	–	+	+	+	+	v	v	–
C. striatum	+	–	–	+	+	+	–	v	v	–

[a]Some or all strains are lipophilic.

Table 5.10 Differential characteristics of nonpigmented coryneform bacteria

Genus	Catalase	Nitrate reductase	Esculin hydrolysis	Other
Oxidative				
Turicella	+	−	−	Long, nonbranching bacilli; CAMP strongly positive
Fermentative				
Dermabacter	+	−	+	Short coccobacilli; pungent odor
Rothia	V	+	+	Pleomorphic cocci and bacilli
Arcanobacterium	−	−	−	Irregular bacilli; reverse CAMP positive
Gardnerella	−	−	−	Gram-variable bacilli or coccobacilli

Table 5.11 Differential characteristics of yellow-pigmented coryneform bacteria

Genus or species	Motility	Nitrate reductase	Hydrolysis of: Casein	Gelatin	Urease	Esulin	Acid from: Glucose	Maltose	Sucrose	Mannitol	Xylose
Oxidative											
Aureobacterium[a]	v	v	+	+	v	v	+	+	v	v	v
Brevibacterium[b]	–	v	+	+	–	–	v	v	v	–	–
"Corynebacterium aquaticum"[c]	+	v	–	–	–	v	+	v	v	+	+
Fermentative											
Microbacterium[d]	v	–	v	v	–	+	+	+	+	+	v
Cellulomonas[e]	v	+	–	+	–	+	+	+	+	v	+
Oerskovia[f]	+	+	+	+	–	+	+	+	+	–	+
Exiguobacterium[g]	+	v	+	v	–	+	+	+	+	+	–

[a]Rapid pigment development; thin bacilli with no branching; catalase variable.
[b]Slow pigment development; coccobacilli to cocci in older cultures; catalase positive; cheesy odor.
[c]Slow pigment development; thin bacilli with no branching; catalase positive.
[d]Coccobacilli; catalase variable; poor anaerobic growth.
[e]Small, thin bacilli; catalase positive; cellulolytic.
[f]Cocci to bacilli with extensive branching; catalase positive; rapid fermentation and esculin reaction.
[g]Coccobacillus; catalase positive.

Microbial Identification

Microbial Identification

Table 5.12 Differential characteristics of selected *Bacillus* species

Species	Growth:			Lecithinase	Casein hydrolysis	Gelatin hydrolysis	Arginine dihydrolase	Acid from:							
	Anaerobic	50°C	60°C					D-Arabinose	Glycerol	Glycogen	Inulin	Mannitol	Salicin
B. anthracis	+	−	−	+	+	+	−	−	−	+	−	−	−
B. cereus	+	−	−	+	+	+	>	−	>	+	−	−	+
B. thuringiensis	+	−	−	+	+	+	+	−	+	+	−	−	+
B. mycoides	+	>	−	+	+	+	>	−	+	+	−	−	+
B. subtilis	−	+	−	−	+	+	−	−	+	+	+	+	+
B. licheniformis	+	−	−	−	+	+	+	−	+	+	>	+	+
B. circulans	+	−	−	−	−	−	−	−	>	+	+	+	+
B. stearothermophilus	−	+	+	+	+	+	−	−	+	+	−	−	−

Table 5.13 Differential characteristics of partially acid-fast organisms: *Nocardia, Rhodococcus, Tsukamurella,* and *Gordona* species

Species	Hydrolysis of: Adenine	Casein	Hypoxanthine	Tyrosine	Xanthine	45°C	0.05% lysozyme broth	Growth: D-Galactose	D-Glucose	D-Sucrose	D-Mannitol	D-Trehalose	D-Sorbitol	L-Rhamnose	i-Erythritol
N. asteroides	-	-	-	-	-	>	+	>	+	NT	-	>	-	-	-
N. farcinica	-	-	-	-	-	+	+	-	+	NT	-	-	-	+	+
N. nova	-	-	-	-	-	-	+	-	+	NT	-	>	-	-	-
N. brevicatena	-	+	-	-	-	>	>	-	-	NT	+	+	-	+	-
N. brasiliensis	-	+	+	+	-	-	+	+	+	NT	+	+	-	-	-
N. pseudobrasiliensis	+	-	+	+	+	-	+	+	+	NT	+	+	-	-	-
N. otitidiscaviarum	-	-	+	-	-	>	+	-	+	NT	>	>	-	-	-
N. transvalensis	-	-	+	-	-	NT	+	>	>	-	>	+	>	-	>
R. equi	+	-	-	-	-	-	>	+	-	NT	-	+	-	>	NT
T. paurometabolum	-	-	-	-	-	-	+	NT	NT	NT	+	NT	+	NT	NT
G. terrae	NT	-	-	-	-	NT	>	-	+	NT	+	+	+	+	NT

Microbial Identification

Table 5.14 Differential characteristics of rapidly growing *Mycobacterium* species

Species	Growth:		Nitrate reductase	Arylsulfatase (3 days)	Iron uptake	Utilization of:			Susceptibility to:	
	MacConkey	5% NaCl				Mannitol	Inositol	Citrate	Polymyxin B	Ciprofloxacin
M. fortuitum	+	+	+	+	+	−	−	−	S	S
M. fortuitum bv. III	+	+	+	+	+	+	−	−	S	S
M. peregrinum	+	+	+	+	+	+	+	−	S	S
M. chelonae	+	−	−	−	+	−	−	+	R	R
M. abscessus	+	+	−	−	+	+	−	−	R	R
M. mucogenicum	+	−	V	−	+	+	−	+	V	S
M. smegmatis	+	+	+	+	−	+	+	V	S	NT

Table 5.15 Differential characteristics of nonchromogenic, slow-growing *Mycobacterium* species

Species	Colony morphology[a]	Niacin	Nitrate reductase	Catalase (>45 mm)	Catalase (68°C)	Tween hydrolysis	Tellurite reduction	Arylsulfatase (3 days)	Urease	Pyrazinamidase
M. tuberculosis	R	+	+	−	−	v	v	−	v	+
M. africanum	R	−	−	−	−	−	−	−	+	−
M. bovis	R	−	−	−	−	v	NT	−	v	−
M. avium complex	S	−	−	+	v	−	+	−	−	+
M. xenopi	S	−	−	−	v	−	v	v	−	v
M. haemophilum	R	−	−	−	−	+	−	−	−	+
M. malmoense	S	−	−	+	v	+	v	−	−	+
M. shimoidei	R	−	−	−	−	+	NT	−	+	+
M. genavense	S	−	−	−	+	+	NT	−	−	+
M. celatum	S	−	−	−	+	−	+	+	v	+
M. ulcerans	R	−	−	−	+	+	NT	−	−	−
M. terrae complex	S/R	−	v	+	+	+	v	v	v	v
M. triviale	R	−	+	+	+	+	v	−	v	v
M. gastri	S/R	−	−	−	−	+	v	−	v	−

[a]R, rough; S, smooth.

Microbial Identification

Microbial Identification

Table 5.16 Differential characteristics of chromogenic, slow-growing *Mycobacterium* species

Species	Pigmentation[a]	Colony morphology[b]	Niacin	Nitrate reductase	Catalase (>45 mm)	Tween hydrolysis	Tolerance to 5% NaCl	Urease	Pyrazinamidase
M. kansasii	P	R/S	−	+	+	+	−	V	−
M. marinum	P	S/R	V	−	−	+	−	+	+
M. simiae	P	S	V	V	+	−	−	V	+
M. asiaticum	P	S	−	−	+	+	−	−	−
M. szulgai	Sc/P	S/R	−	+	+	V	−	V	+
M. xenopi	Sc/N	S	−	−	+	−	−	−	V
M. gordonae	Sc	S	−	−	+	+	−	V	V
M. scrofulaceum	Sc	S	−	−	+	−	−	V	V
M. flavescens	Sc	S	−	+	+	+	V	V	+

[a]P, photochromogen; Sc, scotochromogen; N, nonchromogenic.
[b]R, rough; S, smooth.

Table 5.17 Differential characteristics of non-spore-forming, gram-positive, anaerobic bacilli

Genus	Strict anaerobe	Catalase	Motility	Nitrate reductase	Indole production	Metabolic products (GLC)
Actinomyces	V	−	−	V	−	S, L, a
Bifidobacterium	+	−	−	−	−	A, L
Eubacterium	+	−	V	V	−	(A), (B)
Lactobacillus	V	−	−	−	−	L, (a), (s)
Mobiluncus	+	−	+	V	−	S, A, (L)
Propionibacterium	V	V	−	V	−	A, P, iv, s, l

Microbial Identification

Table 5.18 Differential characteristics of selected *Actinomyces* and *Propionibacterium* species

Species	Catalase	Nitrate reductase	Indole	Urease	Hydrolysis		Acid from:									Metabolic products (GLC)
					Esculin	Gelatin	Glucose	Arabinose	Mannose	Raffinose	Trehalose	Inositol	Glycerol	Xylose	Mannitol	
A. israelii	−	V	−	−	+	−	+	+	+	+	V	+	−	+	+	A, L, S
A. meyeri	−	−	−	+	V	−	+	V	−	−	−	−	V	+	−	A, S
A. naeslundii	−	+	−	+	+	−	+	−	+	+	+	+	V	−	−	A, L, S
A. odontolyticus	−	V	−	−	V	−	+	V	−	−	−	−	V	V	−	A, S
A. pyogenes	−	−	−	−	−	+	+	V	V	−	V	V	V	V	−	A, S
P. acnes	+	+	+	−	−	+	+	−	+	−	−	−	+	−	+	A, P, (iv), (l), (s)
P. propionicus	−	+	−	−	−	+	+	−	V	+	V	V	V	−	V	A, P, (l), (s)

Table 5.19 Differential characteristics of selected *Clostridium* species

| Species | Egg yolk agar | | Gelatinase | Milk digestion | Indole | Acid from: | | | | Metabolic products (GLC) |
	Lecithinase	Lipase				Glucose	Maltose	Lactose	Sucrose	
C. perfringens	+	–	+	–	–	+	+	+	+	A, B, (P), (L)
C. baratii	+	–	–	–	–	+	+	+	+	A, B, (L)
C. novyi A	+	+	+	–	–	+	+	–	–	A, P, B, (V)
C. novyi B	+	–	+	–	–	+	+	–	–	A, P, B
C. novyi C	–	–	V	–	–	+	–	–	–	A, P, B
C. haemolyticum	+	–	+	–	+	+	–	–	–	A, P, B
C. bifermentans	+	–	+	+	+	+	+	–	–	A, IC, (P), (IB), (IV), PP
C. sordellii	+	–	+	+	+	+	+	–	–	A, IC, (P), (IB), (IV)
C. botulinum I	–	+	+	+	–	+	+	–	–	A, IB, B, IV, (P), (V), (IC), PP
C. botulinum II	–	+	+	–	–	+	+	–	+	A, B

(continued)

Microbial Identification

Table 5.19 Differential characteristics of selected *Clostridium* species *(continued)*

Species	Egg yolk agar		Gelatinase	Milk digestion	Indole	Acid from:				Metabolic products (GLC)
	Lecithinase	Lipase				Glucose	Maltose	Lactose	Sucrose	
C. botulinum III	−	+	+	V	−	+	V	−	−	A, P, B
C. sporogenes	−	+	+	+	−	+	+	−	−	A, IB, B, IV, (P), (V), (IC), PP
C. septicum	−	−	+	+	−	+	+	+	+	A, B
C. chauvoei	−	−	+	+	−	+	+	+	−	A, B, F
C. difficile	−	−	+	−	−	+	+	−	−	A, IB, B, IV, V, IC, (P), PP
C. tetani	−	−	+	+	+	−	−	−	−	A, P, B, (PP)
C. histolyticum	−	−	+	−	−	−	−	−	−	A, (PP)
C. sphenoides	−	−	−	−	+	+	+	+	−	A, F
C. tertium	−	−	−	−	+	+	+	+	+	A, B, (L), (PP)
C. butyricum	−	−	−	−	−	+	+	+	+	A, B
C. fallax	−	−	−	−	−	+	+	+	+	A, B, (L)
C. ramosum	−	−	−	−	−	+	+	+	+	A, L, (PY)

Table 5.20 Differential characteristics of selected oxidase-negative, fermentative, gram-negative bacilli

Organism	Growth on MacConkey agar	Catalase	Arginine dihydrolase	Ornithine decarboxylase	Lysine decarboxylase	Urease	Indole production	Nitrate reductase	Acid from: Glucose	Lactose	Sucrose	Mannitol	Maltose	Xylose
Enterobacteriaceae	+	+	V	V	V	V	V	+	+	V	V	V	V	V
Chromobacterium	+	+	+	−	−	V	V	+	+	−	V	−	−	−
Actinobacillus	−	+	−	−	−	−	−	+	+	+	+	V	+	V
Haemophilus aphrophilus	V	−	−	−	−	−	−	+	+	+	+	+	+	−
Capnocytophaga	−	−	−	−	−	−	−	V	+	V	+	−	+	−
DF-3	−	V	−	−	−	−	V	−	+	+	+	−	+	+
Pasteurella multocida	−	+	−	+	−	−	+	+	+	−	+	+	−	V

Microbial Identification

Table 5.21 Differential characteristics of selected members of the *Enterobacteriaceae*

Species	Indole production	Methyl red	Voges-Proskauer	Citrate utilization	Urease	Phenylalanine deaminase	Lysine decarboxylase	Arginine dihydrolase	Ornithine decarboxylase	Motility	Glucose	Lactose	Sucrose	Mannitol	Dulcitol	Adonitol	Maltose	Xylose
											Acid from:							
Citrobacter freundii	V	V	-	V	V	-	-	V	-	+	+	V	+	+	-	-	+	+
Citrobacter koseri	+	+	-	+	V	-	-	V	+	+	+	V	V	+	V	+	+	+
Edwardsiella tarda	+	+	-	-	-	-	+	-	+	+	+	-	-	-	-	-	+	-
Enterobacter aerogenes	-	-	+	+	-	-	+	-	+	+	+	+	+	+	-	+	+	+
Enterobacter cloacae	-	-	+	+	V	-	-	+	+	+	+	+	+	+	V	V	+	+
Escherichia coli	+	+	-	-	-	-	+	V	V	-	+	+	V	+	V	-	+	+
Klebsiella oxytoca	+	V	+	+	+	-	+	-	-	-	+	+	+	+	V	+	+	+
Klebsiella pneumoniae	-	V	+	+	+	-	+	-	-	-	+	+	+	+	V	+	+	+
Morganella morganii	+	+	-	-	+	+	-	-	+	+	+	-	-	-	-	-	-	-

	Proteus mirabilis	*Proteus vulgaris*	*Providencia rettgeri*	*Providencia stuartii*	*Salmonella species*	*Serratia liquefaciens*	*Serratia marcescens*	*Shigella sonnei*	*Yersinia enterocolitica*	*Yersinia pestis*
1	+	+	–	–	+	+	–	–	v	+
2	–	+	–	–	+	+	+	+	v	v
3	–	–	+	–	–	–	v	–	–	–
4	–	–	–	–	+	–	–	–	–	–
5	–	–	+	–	+	+	+	+	+	+
6	v	+	v	+	–	+	+	–	+	–
7	–	–	–	–	–	–	–	–	–	–
8	+	+	+	+	+	+	+	+	+	+
9	+	+	+	v	+	+	+	–	–	–
10	+	–	–	–	+	+	+	+	+	–
11	–	–	–	–	v	–	–	–	–	–
12	–	–	–	–	+	+	+	–	–	–
13	+	+	+	+	–	–	–	–	–	–
14	+	+	+	v	–	–	v	–	v	–
15	v	v	+	+	+	+	+	–	–	–
16	v	–	–	–	–	+	+	–	–	–
17	+	+	+	+	+	+	+	+	+	v
18	–	+	+	+	–	–	–	–	v	–

Microbial Identification

Table 5.22 Differential characteristics of selected oxidase-positive, fermentative, gram-negative bacilli

Genus or species	Growth on MacConkey agar	Catalase	Arginine dihydrolase	Ornithine decarboxylase	Lysine decarboxylase	Urease	Indole production	Nitrate reductase	Acid from: Glucose	Acid from: Lactose	Acid from: Sucrose	Acid from: Mannitol	Acid from: Maltose	Acid from: Xylose
Aeromonas	+								+					
Plesiomonas	+								+					
Vibrio	V								+					
Actinobacillus	–	+	–			–	–	+	+	+	+	V	+	V
Chromobacterium	+	+	+			V	V	+	+	–	V	–	–	–
Haemophilus aphrophilus	V	–	–	–	–	–	–	–	+	+	+	+	+	–
Kingella kingae	–	–	–	–	–	–	–	–	+	–	–	–	+	V
Neisseria	V	+	–	–	–	–	+	+	+	V	V	–	V	V
Pasteurella multocida	–	+		+	–	–	+		+	–	+	+	–	–
Suttonella	V	V		–	–	–	–	V	+	V	+	–	+	–
Capnocytophaga	–	–	NT	–	NT	–			+	–	+	–	+	–
Cardiobacterium	–	–		–		–	+	–	+		+	+	+	–

Table 5.23 Differential characteristics of selected *Vibrio*, *Aeromonas*, and *Plesiomonas* species

Species	Oxidase	Voges-Proskauer	Citrate utilization	Urease	Lysine decarboxylase	Arginine dihydrolase	Ornithine decarboxylase	Acid from: Glucose	Lactose	Sucrose	Salicin	Cellobiose	Arabinose	myo-Inositol	Mannitol
V. cholerae	+	>	+	−	+	−	+	+	−	+	−	−	−	−	+
V. parahaemolyticus	+	−	−	>	+	−	+	+	−	−	−	−	−	−	+
V. vulnificus	+	−	>	−	+	−	+	+	>	>	+	+	−	−	>
V. alginolyticus	+	+	−	−	+	−	+	+	−	+	−	−	−	−	+
A. hydrophila	+	+	>	−	+	+	−	+	−	+	+	>	+	−	+
A. caviae	+	−	>	−	−	+	−	+	+	+	+	+	+	−	+
A. veronii bv. sobria	+	+	>	−	+	+	−	+	−	+	−	>	−	−	+
P. shigelloides	+	−	−	−	+	+	+	+	−	−	>	−	−	+	−

Microbial Identification

Table 5.24 Differential characteristics of *Haemophilus* species

Species	Growth requirement			Hemolysis (horse blood)	Catalase	Acid from:			
	CO$_2$	Hemin (factor X)	NAD (factor V)			Glucose	Sucrose	Lactose	Mannose
H. influenzae	+	+	+	−	+	+	−	−	−
H. aphrophilus	+	+	−	−	−	+	+	+	+
H. haemolyticus	−	+	+	+	+	+	−	−	−
H. parahaemolyticus	−	−	+	+	+	+	+	−	−
H. parainfluenzae	V	−	+	−	V	+	+	−	+
H. paraphrophilus	+	−	+	−	−	+	+	+	+
H. segnis	−	−	+	−	V	+	+	−	−
H. ducreyi	−	+	−	−	−	−	−	−	−

Table 5.25 Differential characteristics of selected oxidase-negative, oxidative, gram-negative bacilli

Genus or species	Growth on MacConkey agar	Catalase	Motility	Arginine dihydrolase	Lysine decarboxylase	Urease	Indole production	Esculin hydrolysis	Nitrate reductase	D-Glucose	OF-lactose	OF-sucrose	OF-mannitol	OF-maltose	OF-xylose
Acinetobacter	+	+	−	V	−	V	−	−	−	+	V	−	−	V	−
Chryseomonas	+	+	+	+	−	V	−	+	V	+	V	V	+	+	+
Flavimonas	+	+	+	V	−	V	−	−	−	+	V	V	+	+	+
Burkholderia cepacia	+	+	+	−	V	V	−	V	V	+	+	V	+	+	+
Roseomonas	+	+	V	−	−	+	−	−	−	V	−	−	V	−	V
Sphingomonas	V	+	V	−	−	−	−	+	−	+	+	+	−	+	+
Stenotrophomonas	+	+	+	−	+	V	−	V	V	+	V	V	−	+	V
Francisella	−	+	NT	−	NT	−	−	NT	−	+	NT	−	NT	−	−

Microbial Identification

Table 5.26 Differential characteristics of selected oxidase-positive, oxidative, gram-negative bacilli

Genus or species	Growth on MacConkey agar	Catalase	Arginine dihydrolase	Lysine decarboxylase	Urease	Indole production	Nitrate reductase	D-Glucose	OF-lactose	OF-sucrose	OF-mannitol	OF-maltose	OF-xylose
Agrobacterium	+	+	-	-	+	-	>	+	+	+	+	+	+
Alcaligenes xylosoxidans	+	+	>	-	-	-	+	>	-	-	-	-	+
Brucella	>	+	-	-	+	-	+	+	-	-	-	-	+
EF-4	>	+	-	-	-	-	+	+	-	-	-	-	-
Chryseobacterium meningosepticum	>	+	-	-	-	+	-	+	>	-	+	+	-
Methylobacterium	>	+	-	-	>	-	>	>	-	-	-	-	+
Ochrobactrum	+	+	>	-	+	-	+	+	-	>	>	>	+
Pseudomonas aeruginosa	+	+	+	-	>	-	+	+	-	-	>	-	+
Pseudomonas fluorescens	+	+	+	-	>	-	>	+	>	>	>	-	+
Burkholderia cepacia	+	+	-	>	>	-	>	+	+	>	+	+	+
Burkholderia pseudomallei	+	+	+	-	>	-	+	+	+	-	+	+	+
Roseomonas	+	+	-	-	+	-	-	>	+	-	>	-	>
Sphingomonas	>	+	-	-	-	-	-	+	-	+	-	+	+
Neisseria gonorrhoeae	-	+	-	NT	-	-	-	+	-	-	-	-	-
Neisseria meningitidis	-	+	-	NT	-	-	-	+	-	-	-	+	-
Neisseria lactamica	-	+	-	NT	-	-	-	+	+	-	-	+	-

Table 5.27 Differential characteristics of the gram-negative bacteria *Neisseria*, *Moraxella*, and *Kingella* species

Species	Growth on[a]: MTM, ML, NYC	CHOC, BA (22°C)	Nutrient agar	Nitrate reductase	DNase	Acid from: Glucose	Maltose	Lactose	Sucrose	Fructose
N. cinerea	V	−	+	−	−	−	−	−	−	−
N. flavescens	−	+	+	−	−	−	−	−	−	−
N. gonorrhoeae	+	−	−	−	−	+	−	−	−	−
N. lactamica	+	V	+	−	−	+	+	+	−	−
N. meningitidis	+	+	V	−	−	+	+	−	−	−
N. mucosa	−	+	+	−	−	+	+	−	V	V
N. polysaccharea	V	+	+	−	−	+	+	−	+	+
N. sicca	−	+	+	−	−	+	+	−	V	V
N. subflava	V	+	+	−	−	+	+	−	−	−
M. catarrhalis	V	+	+	+	+	−	−	−	−	−
K. denitrificans	+	NT	+	+	−	+	−	−	−	−

[a]MTM, modified Thayer-Martin agar; ML, Martin-Lewis agar; NYC, New York City agar; CHOC, chocolate agar; BA, blood agar.

Microbial Identification

Microbial Identification

Table 5.28 Differential characteristics of selected oxidase-negative, nonoxidative, gram-negative bacilli

Genus or species	Growth on MacConkey agar	Motility	Urease	Nitrate reductase	D-Glucose	OF-maltose	OF-xylose
Acinetebacter	V	–	V	–	–	–	–
Bordetella parapertussis	+	–	+	–	–	–	–
Roseomonas	+	V	+	–	–	–	V
Stenotrophomonas	+	–	V	V	+	+	V
Bartonella	–	+	–	–	+	–	–
Francisella	–	–	–	–	+	–	–

Table 5.29 Differential characteristics of selected oxidase-positive, nonoxidative, gram-negative bacilli

Species	Growth on:		Catalase	Motility	Flagella			Urease	Indole production	Nitrate reductase	Nitrate to gas	H₂S on TSI^a	Glucose	OF-mannitol	OF-xylose
	MacConkey agar	SS agar			1–2 polar	>2 polar	Peritrichous								
Afipia felis	>	–	>	+	+	–	–	+	–	+	–	–	–	–	+
Alcaligenes faecalis	+	+	+	+	–	–	+	–	–	–	–	–	–	–	–
Alcaligenes xylosoxidans	+	+	+	+	–	–	+	–	–	+	+	–	–	–	–
Bordetella pertussis	–	–	+	–	–	–	–	+	–	–	–	NT	–	NT	–
Bordetella bronchiseptica	+	+	+	+	–	–	+	+	–	+	–	–	–	–	–
Brucella species	>	–	+	–	–	–	–	+	–	+	>	–	+	–	+
Campylobacter species	>	–	+	+	+	–	–	–	–	+	–	–	–	–	–
Methylobacterium species	>	–	+	+	+	–	–	>	–	>	–	–	>	–	+
Moraxella atlantae	+	–	+	–	–	–	–	–	–	–	–	–	–	–	–
Moraxella catarrhalis	–	–	+	–	–	–	–	–	–	>	–	–	–	–	–
Moraxella osloensis	>	–	+	–	–	–	–	–	–	>	–	–	–	–	–
Moraxella lacunata	–	–	+	–	–	–	–	–	–	–	–	–	–	–	–
Moraxella phenylpyruvica	>	–	+	–	–	–	–	+	–	>	–	–	–	–	–

(continued)

Microbial Identification

Table 5.29 Differential characteristics of selected oxidase-positive, nonoxidative, gram-negative bacilli *(continued)*

Species	Growth on: MacConkey agar	SS agar	Catalase	Motility	Flagella 1–2 polar	<2 polar	Peritrichous	Urease	Indole production	Nitrate reductase	Nitrate to gas	H$_2$S on TSI[a]	Glucose	OF-mannitol	OF-xylose
Neisseria flavescens	V	−	+	−	−	−	−	−	−	−	−	−	−	−	−
Neisseria mucosa	V	−	+	−	−	−	−	−	−	+	+	−	+	−	−
Neisseria sicca	V	−	V	−	−	−	−	−	−	−	−	−	+	−	−
Ochrobactrum anthropi	+	+	+	+	−	−	+	+	−	+	+	V	+	V	+
Oligella ureolytica	V	−	+	V	−	−	V	+	−	+	V	−	−	−	−
Oligella urethralis	+	−	+	−	−	−	−	−	−	−	−	−	−	−	−
Pseudomonas diminuta	+	−	+	+	+	−	−	V	−	−	−	−	V	−	−
Roseomonas species	+	−	+	+	+	−	−	+	−	V	−	−	V	V	V
Bartonella species	−	−	+	−	−	−	−	−	−	−	−	NT	−	−	−
Eikenella corrodens	−	−	−	−	−	−	−	−	−	+	−	−	−	−	−
Kingella denitrificans	−	−	−	−	−	−	−	−	−	+	V	−	+	−	−
Weeksella virosa	−	−	+	−	−	−	−	+	+	+	−	−	−	−	−
Weeksella zoohelcum	−	−	+	−	−	−	−	−	+	−	−	−	−	−	−

[a]TSI, triple sugar iron.

Table 5.30 Differential characteristics of selected *Campylobacter*, *Arcobacter*, and *Helicobacter* species

Species	Catalase	Nitrate reductase	Urease	Alkaline phosphatase	Hippurate hydrolysis	Indoxyl acetate hydrolysis	γ-Glutamyl transferase	Growth: 15°C	25°C	42°C	3.5% NaCl	1% glycine
C. jejuni subsp. jejuni	+	+	−	NT	+	+	NT	−	−	+	−	+
C. coli	+	+	−	NT	−	+	NT	−	−	+	−	+
C. fetus subsp. fetus	+	+	−	NT	−	−	NT	−	+	−	−	+
C. upsaliensis	+	+	−	NT	−	+	NT	−	−	+	−	V
A. butzleri	+	+	−	NT	−	+	NT	+	+	V	V	+
A. cryaerophilus	+	V	−	NT	−	+	NT	+	+	−	−	−
H. pylori	+	−	+	+	−	−	+	−	−	−	−	−
H. cinaedi	+	+	−	−	−	−	−	−	−	−	−	+
H. fennelliae	+	−	−	+	−	+	−	−	−	−	−	+
H. pullorum	+	+	−	−	−	−	NT	−	−	+	−	+

Microbial Identification

Table 5.31 Differential characteristics of anaerobic, gram-negative bacteria

| Species | Susceptibility to: | | | Growth in 20% bile | Formate or fumate required | Nitrate reductase | Indole | Catalase | Lipase | Urease |
	Kanamycin (1,000 µg)	Vancomycin (5 µg)	Colistin (10 µg)							
Bacteroides fragilis group	R	R	R	+	–	–	>	>	–	–
Other *Bacteroides* spp.	R	R	>	>	–	–	>	>	–	–
Porphyromonas spp.[a]	R	S	R	–	–	–	+	–	–	–
Prevotella spp.[a]	R	R	>	–	–	–	>	–	>	–
Bilophila wadsworthia	S	R	S	+	–	+	–	+	–	+
Fusobacterium nucleatum	S	R	S	–	–	–	+	–	–	–
Other *Fusobacterium* spp.	S	R	S	>	–	–	>	–	>	–
Acidaminococcus fermentans	S	R	S	–	–	–	–	–	–	–
Megasphaera elsdenii	S	R	S	–	–	–	–	–	–	–
Veillonella spp.	S	R	S	–	–	+	–	>	–	–

[a]*Porphyromonas* and some *Prevotella* spp. initially fluoresce red and then develop pigmented colonies.

Table 5.32 Differential characteristics of the *Bacteroides fragilis* group

Species	Indole	Catalase	Esculin hydrolysis	α-Fucosidase	Acid from:							Metabolic products (GLC)
					Arabinose	Cellobiose	Rhamnose	Salicin	Sucrose	Trehalose	Xylan	
B. fragilis	−	+	+	+	−	>	−	−	+	−	−	A, p, S, pa (ib, iv, l)
B. caccae	−	>	+	+	+	>	>	>	+	+	−	A, p, S (iv)
B. distasonis	−	>	+	−	>	+	>	+	+	+	−	A, p, S (pa, ib, iv, l)
B. merdae	−	>	+	−	>	>	+	+	+	+	>	A, p, S (ib, iv)
B. vulgatus	−	>	>	+	+	−	+	−	+	−	>	A, p, S
B. thetaiotaomicron	+	+	+	+	+	>	+	>	+	+	−	A, p, S, pa (ib, iv, l)
B. eggerthii	+	−	+	−	+	>	>	−	−	−	+	A, p, S (ib, iv, l)
B. ovatus	+	>	+	+	+	+	+	+	+	+	+	A, p, S, pa (ib, iv, l)
B. stercoris	+	−	>	>	>	>	+	>	+	−	>	A, p, S, f (ib, iv)
B. uniformis	+	>	+	+	+	+	>	>	+	−	>	a, p, l, S (ib, iv)

Microbial Identification

Microbial Identification

Table 5.33 Differential characteristics of fermentative yeasts[a]

Species	Assimilation tests												Fermentation tests						Urease
	Glucose	Maltose	Sucrose	Lactose	Galactose	Melibiose	Cellobiose	Inositol	Xylose	Raffinose	Trehalose	Dulcitol	Glucose	Maltose	Sucrose	Lactose	Galactose	Trehalose	
Candida albicans	+	+	v	−	+	−	−	−	+	−	+	−	+	+	−	−	+	+	−
Candida catenulata	+	+	−	−	+	−	−	−	+	−	−	−	v	−	−	−	−	−	−
Candida glabrata	+	−	−	−	−	−	−	−	−	−	+	−	+	−	−	−	−	+	−
Candida guilliermondii	+	+	+	+	+	+	+	−	+	+	+	+	+	+	+	−	v	+	−
Candida kefyr	+	−	+	+	+	−	v	−	v	+	v	−	+	−	+	v	+	−	−
Candida krusei	+	−	−	−	−	−	−	−	+	−	−	−	+	−	−	−	−	−	v
Candida lambica	+	−	−	−	−	−	−	−	−	−	−	−	−	−	−	−	−	−	−
Candida lipolytica	+	−	−	−	−	−	+	−	+	−	−	−	+	−	−	−	−	−	+
Candida lusitaniae	+	+	+	−	+	−	−	−	+	−	+	−	−	−	+	−	+	+	−
Candida parapsilosis	+	+	+	−	+	−	−	−	+	−	+	−	+	−	−	−	−	−	−
Candida pintolopesii	+	−	−	−	−	−	−	−	−	−	−	−	+	−	−	−	−	−	−
Candida rugosa	+	−	−	−	+	−	+	−	v	−	−	−	+	−	−	−	−	+	−
Candida tropicalis	+	+	+	−	+	−	v	−	+	−	+	−	+	+	+	−	+	−	−
Candida zeylanoides	+	+	−	−	v	−	−	−	+	+	+	−	−	−	+	−	+	−	−
Saccharomyces cerevisiae	+	+	+	−	+	−	+	−	−	+	v	−	+	+	+	−	+	v	−
Hansenula anomala	+	+	+	−	+	−	+	−	+	−	+	−	+	v	+	−	+	−	−

[a]The morphology on cornmeal agar must be consistent with the biochemical identification. Strain variations will be observed in individual reactions.

Microbial Identification   213

Table 5.34 Differential characteristics of nonfermentative yeasts and yeast-like organisms[a]

	Assimilation tests												Urease
Species	Glucose	Maltose	Sucrose	Lactose	Galactose	Melibiose	Cellobiose	Inositol	Xylose	Raffinose	Trehalose	Dulcitol	
Cryptococcus neoformans	+	+	+	−	+	−	+	+	+	>	+	+	+
Cryptococcus albidus	+	+	+	>	>	+	+	+	+	+	+	>	+
Cryptococcus laurentii	+	+	+	+	+	>	+	+	+	>	+	+	+
Cryptococcus luteolus	+	>	+	−	+	+	+	+	+	+	+	+	+
Cryptococcus terreus	+	+	−	>	>	−	>	+	+	−	>	−	+
Cryptococcus uniguttulatus	+	+	+	−	>	−	+	+	+	>	+	−	+
Rhodotorula glutinis	+	+	+	−	>	−	+	−	+	+	+	−	+
Rhodotorula rubra	+	+	+	−	+	−	>	−	+	+	+	−	+
Geotrichum candidum	+	−	−	−	+	−	−	−	+	−	−	−	−
Blastoschizomyces capitatus	+	−	−	−	+	−	−	−	−	−	−	−	−
Prototheca wickerhamii	+	−	−	−	+	−	−	−	−	−	+	−	−

[a]The morphology on cornmeal agar must be consistent with the biochemical identification. Strain variations will be observed in these reactions.

Microbial Identification

Identification of Filamentous Fungi

Thermally Dimorphic Fungi

1. *Blastomyces dermatitidis:* small microconidia attached to conidiophores or thin hyphae; large, thick-walled, broad-based, budding yeasts at 37°C
2. *Histoplasma capsulatum:* individual pear-shaped microconidia and large tuberculate macroconidia; small, oval budding yeasts at 37°C
3. *Paracoccidioides brasiliensis:* intercalary and terminal chlamydospores on septated hyphae with rare microconidia; large cells with multiple buds at 37°C ("ship's wheel")
4. *Penicillium marneffei:* red colony and reverse; typical *Penicillium* structure at 25–30°C; round or oval yeasts at 37°C
5. *Sporothrix schenckii:* thin septated hyphae with ovoid conidia in rosettes or individually on sides of older hyphae; oval and fusiform yeasts at 37°C

Thermally Monomorphic Fungi

1. White, cream, or light gray surface; nonpigmented reverse
   a. With microconidia or macroconidia
      Acremonium: dematiaceous; long, narrow phialides with large cluster of single, oblong conidia at apices
      Beauveria: hyaline hyphae; conidiogenous cells with swollen bases and zigzagging apices; oval, pale conidia
      Chrysosporium: hyaline hyphae; 45° branching; solitary, unicellular, pyriform conidia at ends of short pedicels or hyphae; arthroconidia in short chains
      Emmonsia: hyaline hyphae; conidiophores branch at right angles; round, unicellular conidia; reactive in *Blastomyces* antigen and probe tests
      Fusarium: hyaline hyphae; cylindrical phialides; ovoid, unicellular or bicellular microconidia; multicellular, curved macroconidia
      Microsporum: dermatophyte; many species; large, rough-walled macroconidia; small, pyriform or clavate microconidia usually arranged singly along hyphae
      Pseudallescheria: hyaline hyphae; brown cleistothecia with ellipsoidal yellow to brown ascospores

Sepedonium: hyaline hyphae; single, rounded, echinulate conidia; resembles *Histoplasma* spp.; distinguished by rapid growth and absence of microaleurioconidia

Stachybotrys: hyaline hyphae; ellipsoidal phialides grouped 3–10 at tips of conidiophores; black, unicellular, ellipsoidal conidia massed at apices of phialides

Trichophyton: dermatophyte; many species; produce large, smooth-walled macroconidia and small, globose, pyriform, or clavate microconidia; microconidia typically most numerous

Verticillium: hyaline hyphae; long, narrow phialides grouped around conidiophore; ovoid, unicellular conidia clustered at tips of phialides

b. Having sporangia or sporangiola; broad, nonseptated, hyaline hyphae

Absidia: pear-shaped apophysis beneath sporangium; rhizoids not at base

Basidiobolus: sporangiophores inflated apically; with ballistospores

Conidiobolus: sporangiophores not inflated; with ballistospores

Cunninghamella: individual spores form on surface of round vesicle

Mucor: branched sporangiophores; no apophysis or rhizoids

Rhizomucor: branched sporangiophores; no apophysis, rhizoids not at base

Rhizopus: sporangiophores single or in clusters; rhizoids at base

Saksenaea: flask-shaped sporangia with elongated sporangiospores; rhizoids near base

c. Having arthroconidia

Coccidioides: hyaline hyphae; no conidiophores; unicellular, barrel-shaped arthroconidia separated by empty cells (disjunctors); spherules with endospores in tissue

Geotrichum: hyaline hyphae; no conidiophores; rectangular arthroconidia; no disjunctors

d. Having only hyphae with chlamydoconidia

Microsporum (see 1a)

Trichophyton (see 1a)

2. White, cream, beige, or light gray surface; yellow, orange, or reddish reverse

Acremonium (see 1a)

Chaetomium: hyaline hyphae; round, brown to black perithecia with brown, lemon-shaped ascospores

Microsporum (see 1a)

Trichophyton (see 1a)

3. White, cream, beige, or light gray surface; red to purple reverse

Microsporum (see 1a)

Penicillium: hyaline hyphae; phialides in brush-like clusters at ends of simple or branched conidiophores; round to ovoid conidia in chains

Trichophyton (see 1a)

4. White, cream, beige, or light gray surface; brown reverse

Chaetomium (see 2)

Chrysosporium (see 1a)

Emmonsia (see 1a)

Madurella: dematiaceous; usually sterile; chlamydospores or vase-shaped phialides occasionally observed

Microsporum (see 1a)

Scopulariopsis: hyaline hyphae; conidiophores with annellides; unicellular, round conidia in chains

Sporotrichum: hyaline hyphae; short conidiophores with single-celled, ovoid conidia

Trichophyton (see 1a)

5. White, cream, beige, or light gray surface; black reverse

Chaetomium (see 2)

Graphium (see 1a)

Nigrospora: hyaline hyphae; short, swollen conidiophores; black, unicellular, ovoid conidia

Phoma: dematiaceous; round, brown to black pycnda with pale, ellipsoidal conidia

Pseudallescheria (see 1a)

Scedosporium: asexual stage of *Pseudallescheria*; hyaline hyphae; conidiophores with simple annellides; pale brown, unicellular, ovoid conidia at ends of conidiophores or on hyphae; cleistothecia occasionally seen

Trichophyton (see 1a)

6. Tan to brown surface

a. Having small conidia

Aspergillus: many species; hyaline hyphae; basal foot cell in hyphae; conidiophores terminate in api-

Microbial Identification

cal vesicle; phialides attached directly to vesicle or bridged with metjula cell; conidia in chains

Botrytis: hyaline hyphae; large, branched conidiophores terminating in vesicles; oval blastoconidia clustered at apices

Chrysosporium (see 1a)

Cladosporium: dematiaceous; brown conidiophores with chains of oval, brown blastoconidia

Dactylaria: dematiaceous; erect conidiophores with constricted, bent point at attachment of bicellular, oval conidia

Emmonsia (see 1a)

Paecilomyces: hyaline hyphae; branched conidiophores; thin, elongated phialides with long chains of oval conidia

Phialophora: dematiaceous; bottle-shaped phialides with collarette at tip; brown, unicellular, oval conidia that accumulate at tip of phialides

Pseudallescheria (see 1a)

Scopulariopsis (see 4)

Sporotrichum (see 4)

Trichophyton (see 1a)

Verticillium (see 1a)

b. Having large conidia or sporangia

Alternaria: dematiaceous; brown, septated conidiophores; brown, muriform, ovoid or obclavate conidia in chains or singly

Basidiobolus (see 1b)

Bipolaris: dematiaceous; brown conidiophores with clusters of five or more fusiform, multiseptated conidia

Botrytis (see 6a)

Conidiobolus (see 1b)

Curvularia: dematiaceous; brown, septated conidiophores; slightly curved, brown, multiseptated poroconidia; central cell larger and darker

Epicoccum: dematiaceous; short conidiophores grouped in clusters; brown, muriform, rounded conidia

Epidermophyton: dermatophyte with smooth-walled, clavate macroconidia in clusters of two or three; no microconidia

Fusarium (see 1a)

Microsporum (see 1a)

Rhizomucor (see 1b)

Rhizopus (see 1b)

Trichophyton (see 1a)

Ulocladium: dematiaceous; geniculate, brown conidiophores; brown, muriform conidia produced singly or (uncommonly) in short chains

   c. Having miscellaneous microscopic morphology

Chaetomium (see 2)

Coccidioides (see 1c)

Madurella (see 4)

Phoma (see 5)

7. Yellow to orange surface

Aspergillus (see 6a)

Chrysosporium (see 1a)

Epicoccum (see 6b)

Epidermophyton (see 6b)

Microsporum (see 1a)

Penicillium (see 3)

Sepedonium (see 1a)

Sporotrichum (see 4)

Trichophyton (see 1a)

Trichothecium: hyaline hyphae; unbranched conidiophores; two-celled, club-shaped conidia arranged in an alternating column at end of conidiophore

Verticillium (see 1a)

8. Pink to violet surface

Acremonium (see 1a)

Aspergillus (see 6a)

Chrysosporium (see 1a)

Fusarium (see 1a)

Microsporum (see 1a)

Paecilomyces (see 6a)

Sporotrichum (see 4)

Trichophyton (see 1a)

Verticillium (see 1a)

9. Green surface; light reverse

Aspergillus (see 6a)

Epidermophyton (see 6b)

Penicillium (see 3)

Trichoderma: hyaline hyphae; branched conidiophores; clusters of round, green conidia at ends of phialides

Verticillium (see 1a)

10. Dark gray or black surface; light reverse

Aspergillus (see 6a)

11. Green, dark gray, or black surface; dark reverse
   a. Having small conidia

   Aureobasidium: dematiaceous hyphae; brown chlamydospores or arthroconidia; with pale blastoconidia

   Botrytis (see 6a)

   Cladosporium (see 6a)

   Exophiala: dematiaceous; cylindrical annellides with pointed tip; brown, oval conidia clustered at tip of annellide or along length

   Fonsecaea: dematiaceous; cylindrical conidiophorese with inflated tip; unicellular, round to ellipsoidal blastoconidia at tips

   Phialophora (see 6a)

   Pseudallescheria (see 1a)

   Scedosporium (see 5)

   Wangiella: dematiaceous; conidiophores not differentiated from hyphae; brown, ellipsoidal phialides with brown, unicellular, oval conidia at tips

   Xylohypha: dematiaceous; brown, septated conidiophores not differentiated from hyphae; long chains of brown, ellipsoidal, unicellular conidia

   b. Having large conidia

   Alternaria (see 6b)

   Bipolaris (see 6b)

   Curvularia (see 6b)

   Dactylaria (see 6a)

   Epicoccum (see 6b)

   Helminthosporium: dematiaceous; brown conidiophores with obclavate, multiseptated poroconidia along perimeter

   Nigrospora (see 5)

   Pithomyces: dematiaceous; undifferentiated conidiophores with single, brown, muriform, club-shaped conidia

   Stachybotrys (see 1a)

   Stemphylium (see 6b)

   Ulocladium (see 6b)

   c. Having only hyphae

   Madurella (see 4)

   d. Having large fruiting bodies

   Chaetomium (see 2)

   Phoma (see 5)

Microbial Identification

Table 5.35 Trophozoites of common intestinal amebae

Organism	Size[a] (diam or length)	Motility	Nucleus (no. and visibility)	Appearance of stained:			
				Peripheral chromatin	Karyosome	Cytoplasm	Inclusions
Entamoeba histolytica	5–60 μm; usual range, 15–20 μm; invasive forms may be >20 μm	Progressive, with hyaline, fingerlike pseudopodia; may be rapid	1; difficult to see in unstained preparations	Fine granules, uniform in size and usually evenly distributed; may appear beaded	Small, usually compact; centrally located but may also be eccentric	Finely granular, "ground glass"; clear differentiation of ectoplasm and endoplasm; if present, vacuoles are usually small	Noninvasive organism may contain bacteria; erythrocytes, if present, are diagnostic
Entamoeba hartmanni	5–12 μm; usual range, 8–10 μm	Usually nonprogressive	1; usually not seen in unstained preparations	Nucleus may stain more darkly than that of *E. histolytica*, although morphology is similar; chromatin may appear as solid ring rather than beaded	Usually small and compact; may be centrally located or eccentric	Finely granular	May contain bacteria; no erythrocytes

	Size	Motility	No. of nuclei	Peripheral chromatin	Karyosomal chromatin	Cytoplasm appearance	Inclusions
Entamoeba coli	15–50 μm; usual range, 20–25 μm	Sluggish, nondirectional, with blunt, granular pseudopodia	1; often visible in unstained preparations	May be clumped and unevenly arranged on membrane; may also appear as solid dark ring with no beads or clumps	Large, not compact; may or may not be eccentric; may be diffuse and darkly stained	Granular, with little differentiation into ectoplasm and endoplasm; usually vacuolated	Bacteria, yeast cells, other debris
Endolimax nana	6–12 μm; usual range, 8–10 μm	Sluggish, usually nonprogressive	1; occasionally visible in unstained preparations	Usually no peripheral chromatin; nuclear chromatin may be quite variable	Large, irregularly shaped; may appear "blotlike"; many nuclear variations are common; may mimic *E. hartmanni* or *Dientamoeba fragilis*	Granular, vacuolated	Bacteria
Iodamoeba bütschlii	8–20 μm; usual range, 12–15 μm	Sluggish, usually nonprogressive	1; usually not visible in unstained preparations	Usually no peripheral chromatin	Large; may be surrounded by refractile granules that are difficult to see ("basket nucleus")	Coarsely granular; may be highly vacuolated	Bacteria, yeast cells, other debris

[a]Wet-preparation measurements (in permanent stains, organisms usually measure 1 to 2 μm less).

Source: L. S. Garcia and D. A. Bruckner, *Diagnostic Medical Parasitology*, 3rd ed., American Society for Microbiology, Washington, D.C., 1997.

Microbial Identification

Microbial Identification

Table 5.36 Cysts of common intestinal amebae

Organism	Size[a] (diam or length)	Shape	Nucleus (no. and visibility)	Appearance of stained: Peripheral chromatin	Karyosome	Cytoplasm, chromatoidal bodies	Glycogen[b]
Entamoeba histolytica	10–20 μm; usual range, 12–15 μm	Usually spherical	Mature cyst, 4; immature, 1 or 2; characteristics difficult to see on wet preparation	Fine, uniform granules, evenly distributed; nuclear characteristics may not be as clearly visible as in trophozoite	Small, compact, usually centrally located but occasionally eccentric	May be present; bodies usually elongate with blunt, rounded, smooth edges; may be round or oval	May be diffuse or absent in mature cyst; clumped chromatin mass may be present in early cysts
Entamoeba hartmanni	5–10 μm; usual range, 6–8 μm	Usually spherical	Mature cyst, 4; immature, 1 or 2; 2 nucleated cysts very common	Fine granules evenly distributed on membrane; nuclear characteristics may be difficult to see	Small, compact, usually centrally located	Usually present; bodies usually elongate with blunt, rounded, smooth edges; may be round or oval	May or may not be present, as in *E. histolytica*
Entamoeba coli	10–35 μm; usual range, 15–25 μm	Usually spherical; may be oval, triangular, or other; may be	Mature cyst, 8; occasionally ≥16; immature cysts with ≥2 nuclei	Coarsely granular; may be clumped and unevenly arranged on	Large, may or may not be compact and/or eccentric; occasionally	May be present (less frequently than in *E. histolytica*); splinter shaped	May be diffuse or absent in mature cyst; clumped mass occasionally

	distorted on permanent stained slide owing to inadequate fixative penetration	occasionally seen	membrane; nuclear characteristics not as clearly defined as in trophozoite; may resemble *E. histolytica*	centrally located	with rough, pointed ends	seen in mature cysts
Endolimax nana	5–10 μm; usual range, 6–8 μm	Usually oval; may be round	Mature cyst, 4; immature cysts, 2, very rarely seen and may resemble cysts of *Enteromonas hominis*	Rarely present; small granules or inclusions are occasionally seen; fine linear chromatoidal bodies may be faintly visible on well-stained smears	Smaller than karyosome seen in trophozoites but generally larger than those of genus *Entamoeba*	No peripheral chromatin	Usually diffuse if present
Iodamoeba bütschlii	5–20 μm; usual range, 10–12 μm	May vary from oval to round; cyst may collapse owing to large glycogen vacuole space	Mature cyst, 1	No peripheral chromatin	Larger, usually eccentric refractile granules may be on one side of karyosome ("basket nucleus")	None; small granules are occasionally present	Large, compact, well-defined mass

[a] Wet-preparation measurements (in permanent stains, organisms usually measure 1 to 2 μm less).
[b] Stains reddish brown with iodine.
Source: L. S. Garcia and D. A. Bruckner, *Diagnostic Medical Parasitology,* 3rd ed., American Society for Microbiology, Washington, D.C., 1997.

Microbial Identification

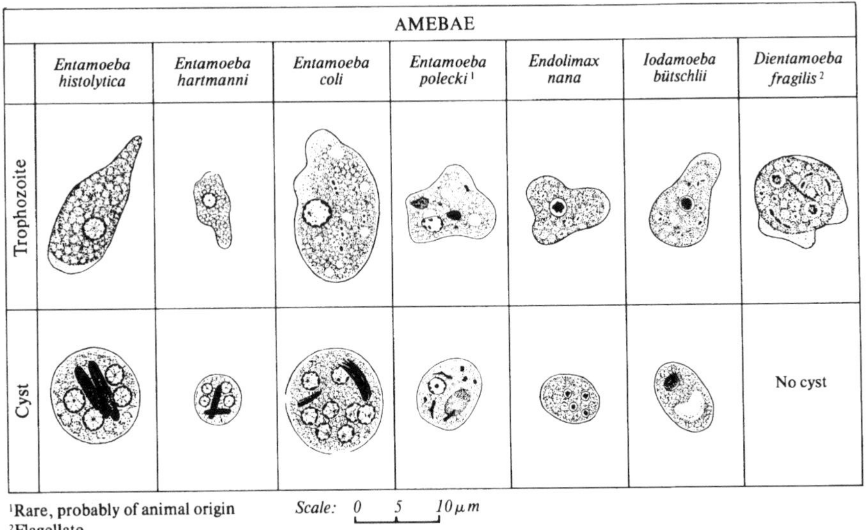

Microbial Identification

Figure 5.1 Amebae and flagellate (*Dientamoeba fragilis*) found in human stool specimens. From M. Brooke and D. Melvin, *Morphology of Diagnostic Stages of Intestinal Parasites of Humans*, 2nd ed., U.S. Department of Health and Human Services publication no. (CDC) 84-8116, Centers for Disease Control and Prevention, Atlanta, Ga., 1984.

Table 5.37 Morphological characteristics of ciliates, coccidia, and tissue protozoa

Species	Shape and size	Other features[a]
Balantidium coli	Trophozoite: ovoid with tapering anterior; 50–100 µm long; 40–70 µm wide (usual width range, 40–50 µm) Cyst: spherical or oval; 50–70 µm in diam (usual range, 50–55 µm)	Trophozoite: 1 large, kidney-shaped macronucleus; 1 small, round micronucleus, which is difficult to see even in stained smears; macronucleus may be visible in unstained preparations; body is covered with cilia, which tend to be longer near cytostome; cytoplasm may be vacuolated Cyst: 1 large macronucleus visible in unstained preparations; micronucleus difficult to see; macronucleus and contractile vacuoles are visible in young cysts; in older cysts, internal structure appears granular; cilia difficult to see within cyst wall
Cryptosporidium parvum	Oocyst generally round, 4–5 µm in diam; each mature oocyst contains sporozoites, which may or may not be visible	Oocyst is the usual diagnostic stage in stool. Various other stages in life cycle can be seen in biopsy specimens taken from GI tract (brush borders of epithelial cells in intestinal tract) and other tissues (respiratory tract, biliary tract).
Cyclospora cayetanensis	Organisms generally round, 8–9 µm in diam; acid-fast like *Cryptosporidium* spp., but larger	Resemble nonrefractile spheres in wet-preparation smears; autofluoresce with epifluorescence; stain variably with acid-fast stains; appear clear, round, and somewhat wrinkled in trichrome stains
Isospora belli	Ellipsoidal oocyst; usual size, 20–30 µm long, 10–19 µm wide; sporocysts rarely seen out of oocysts but measure 9–11 µm	Mature oocyst contains 2 sporocysts with 4 sporozoites each; immature oocysts are usually seen in fecal specimens.

(continued)

Microbial Identification

Table 5.37 Morphological characteristics of ciliates, coccidia, and tissue protozoa (*continued*)

Species	Shape and size	Other features[a]
Microsporidia	Spores are extremely small and have been recovered from all body organs.	Histology results vary; acid-fast, trichrome, and calcofluor white stains recommended for spores. Animal inoculation not recommended. Enteric infections in AIDS patients difficult to diagnose by examining stool specimens.
Pneumocystis carinii	Trophozoite: ameboid shape; about 5 μm long; nucleus visible with Giemsa or hematoxylin stain Cyst: usually round; when mature, contains 8 trophozoites; often 5 μm in diam and contains very small (1-μm) trophozoites	Diagnosis of infections is based on microscopic observation of trophozoites or cysts in clinical (e.g., respiratory) specimens.
Toxoplasma gondii	Trophozoite (tachyzoite): crescent shaped; 4–6 μm long by 2–3 μm wide Cyst (bradyzoite): generally spherical; 200 μm to 1 mm in diam	Diagnosis is most frequently based on clinical history and serologic evidence of infection.
Sarcocystis spp.	Oocyst with thin wall contains 2 mature sporocysts, each containing 4 sporozoites; oocyst frequently ruptures; ovoid sporocysts, each 9–16 μm long and 7.5–12 μm wide	Thin-walled oocyst or ovoid sporocysts occur in stool.

[a]GI, gastrointestinal; PAS, periodic acid-Schiff.

Source: L. S. Garcia and D. A. Bruckner. *Diagnostic Medical Parasitology*, 3rd ed., American Society for Microbiology, Washington, D.C., 1997.

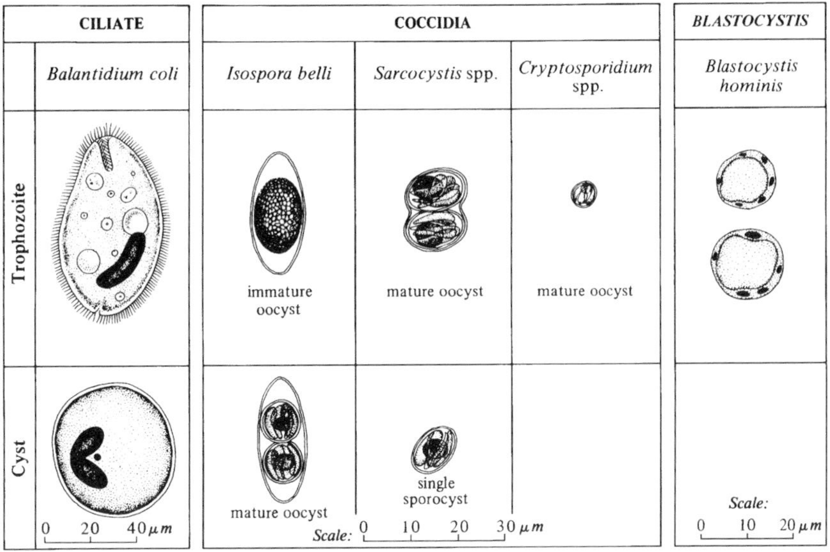

Figure 5.2 Ciliate, coccidia, and *Blastocystis hominis* found in human stool specimens. From M. Brooke and D. Melvin, *Morphology of Diagnostic Stages of Intestinal Parasites of Humans*, 2nd ed., U.S. Department of Health and Human Services publication no. (CDC) 84-8116, Centers for Disease Control and Prevention, Atlanta, Ga., 1984.

Microbial Identification

Microbial Identification

Table 5.38 Trophozoites of flagellates

Organism	Shape and size	Motility	Nucleus (no. and visibility)	No. of flagella[a]	Other features
Dientamoeba fragilis	Shaped like amebae; 5–15 μm (usual range, 9–12 μm)	Usually nonprogressive; pseudopodia are angular, serrated, or broad lobed and almost transparent	Percentage may vary, but 40% of organisms have 1 nucleus and 60% have 2 nuclei; not visible in unstained preparations; no peripheral chromatin; karyosome is cluster of 4–8 granules	No visible flagella	Cytoplasm finely granular and may be vacuoled with ingested bacteria, yeasts, and other debris; may be great variation in size and shape on single smear
Giardia lamblia	Pear shaped; 10–20 μm long; 5–15 μm wide	Falling-leaf motility may be difficult to see if organism is in mucus	2; not visible in unstained mounts	4 lateral, 2 ventral, 2 caudal	Sucking disk occupying 1/2–3/4 of ventral surface; pear shaped from front, spoon shaped from side

Chilomastix mesnili	Pear shaped; 6–24 μm long (usual range, 10–15 μm long), 4–8 μm wide	Stiff, rotary	1; not visible in unstained mounts	3 anterior, 1 in cytostome	Prominent cytostome extending 1/3–1/2 length of body; spiral groove across ventral surface
Trichomonas hominis	Pear shaped; 5–15 μm long (usual range, 7–9 μm long), 7–10 μm wide	Jerky, rapid	1; not visible in unstained mounts	3–5 anterior, 1 posterior	Undulating membrane extends length of body; posterior flagellum extends free beyond end of body
Trichomonas tenax	Pear shaped; 5–12 μm long (usual range, 6.5–7.5 μm), 7–9 μm wide	Jerky, rapid	1; not visible in unstained mounts	4 anterior, 1 posterior	Seen only in preparations from mouth; axostyle (slender rod) protrudes beyond posterior end and may be visible; posterior flagellum extends only halfway down body, and there is no free end

(continued)

Microbial Identification

Table 5.38 Trophozoites of flagellates *(continued)*

Organism	Shape and size	Motility	Nucleus (no. and visibility)	No. of flagella[a]	Other features
Trichomonas vaginalis	Pear shaped; 7–23 μm long (usual range, 13 μm), 5–15 μm wide	Jerky, rapid	1; not visible in unstained mounts	3–5 anterior; 1 posterior	Undulating membrane extends 1/2 length of body; no free posterior flagellum; axostyle easily seen
Enteromonas hominis	Oval, 4–10 μm long (usual range, 8–9 μm long), 5–6 μm wide	Jerky	1; not visible in unstained mounts	3 anterior, 1 posterior	One side of body flattened; posterior flagellum extends free posteriorly or laterally
Retortamonas intestinalis	Pear shaped or oval; 4–9 μm long (usual range, 6–7 μm long), 3–4 μm wide	Jerky	1; not visible in unstained mounts	1 anterior, 1 posterior	Prominent cytostome extending approximately 1/2 length of body

[a]Usually difficult to see.

Source: L. S. Garcia and D. A. Bruckner, *Diagnostic Medical Parasitology*, 3rd ed., American Society for Microbiology, Washington, D.C., 1997.

Table 5.39 Cysts of flagellates[a]

Species	Size	Shape	Nuclei (no. and visibility)	Other features
Dientamoeba fragilis, Trichomonas hominis, Trichomonas tenax	No cyst stage	NA	NA	NA
Giardia lamblia	8–19 µm long (usual range, 11–14 µm long), 7–10 µm wide	Oval, ellipsoidal, or round	4; not distinct in unstained preparations; usually located at one end	Longitudinal fibers in cysts may be visible in unstained preparations; deeply staining median bodies usually lie across longitudinal fibers; there is often shrinkage, and cytoplasm pulls away from cyst wall; may also be "halo" effect around outside of cyst wall due to shrinkage caused by dehydrating reagents

(continued)

Microbial Identification

Table 5.39 Cysts of flagellates[a] (continued)

Species	Size	Shape	Nuclei (no. and visibility)	Other features
Chilomastix mesnili	6–10 μm long (usual range, 7–9 μm long), 4–6 μm wide	Lemon shaped with anterior hyaline knob	1; not distinct in unstained preparations	Cytostome with supporting fibrils, usually visible in stained preparation; curved fibril alongside of cytostome usually referred to as "shepherd's crook"
Enteromonas hominis	4–10 μm long (usual range, 6–8 μm long), 4–6 μm wide	Elongate or oval	1–4; usually 2 lying at opposite ends of cyst; not visible in unstained mounts	Resembles *Endolimax nana* cyst; fibrils or flagella usually not seen
Retortamonas intestinalis	4–9 μm long (usual range, 4–7 μm long), 5 μm wide	Pear shaped or slightly lemon shaped	1; not visible in unstained mounts	Resembles *Chilomastix* cyst; shadow outline of cytostome with supporting fibrils extends above nucleus; bird beak fibril arrangement

[a]NA, not applicable.
Source: L. S. García and D. A. Bruckner, *Diagnostic Medical Parasitology*, 3rd ed., American Society for Microbiology, Washington, D.C., 1997.

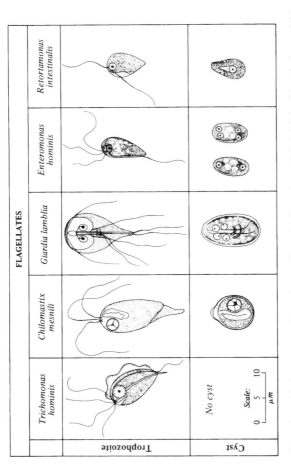

Figure 5.3 Flagellates found in human stool specimens. From M. Brooke and D. Melvin, *Morphology of Diagnostic Stages of Intestinal Parasites of Humans*, 2nd ed., U.S. Department of Health and Human Services publication no. (CDC) 84-8116, Centers for Disease Control and Prevention, Atlanta, Ga., 1984.

Microbial Identification

Microbial Identification

Table 5.40 Morphological characteristics of parasites found in blood[a]

Organism	Diagnostic stage
Malaria parasites	
Plasmodium vivax (benign tertian malaria)	Amoeboid rings; presence of Schüffner's dots; all stages seen in peripheral blood; mature schizont contains 16–18 merozoites; infects young RBCs
Plasmodium ovale (ovale malaria)	Nonameboid rings; presence of Schüffner's dots; all stages seen in peripheral blood; mature schizont contains 8–10 merozoites; RBCs may be oval and have fimbriated edges; infects young RBCs
Plasmodium malariae (quartan malaria)	Rings are thick; no stippling; all stages seen in peripheral blood; presence of band forms and rosette-shaped mature schizont; lots of malarial pigment; infects mature RBCs
Plasmodium falciparum (malignant tertian malaria)	Multiple rings; appliqué/accolé forms; no stippling (rare Maurer's clefts); rings and crescent-shaped gametocytes seen in peripheral blood (no other developing stages, with rare exception of mature schizont); infects all RBCs
Babesia spp.	Ring forms only (resemble *P. falciparum* rings); seen in splenectomized patients; endemic in the United States (no travel history necessary); if present, "Maltese cross" configuration diagnostic
Trypanosoma brucei gambiense (West African sleeping sickness)	Trypomastigotes long and slender, with typical undulating membrane; lymph nodes and blood can be sampled; microhematocrit tube concentration helpful; examine spinal fluid in later stages of infection
Trypanosoma brucei rhodesiense (East African sleeping sickness)	Trypomastigotes long and slender, with typical undulating membrane; lymph nodes and blood can be sampled; microhematocrit tube concentration helpful; examine spinal fluid in later stages of infection
Trypanosoma cruzi (Chagas' disease, South American trypanosomiasis)	Trypomastigotes short and stumpy, often curved in C shape; blood sampled early in infection; trypomastigotes enter striated muscle (heart, GI tract) and transform into amastigote form
Leishmania spp. (cutaneous; not actually a blood parasite but presented for comparison with *Leishmania donovani*)	Amastigotes found in macrophages of skin; presence of intracellular forms containing nucleus and kinetoplast diagnostic

Leishmania braziliensis (mucocutaneous; not actually a blood parasite but presented for comparison with *Leishmania donovani*)	Amastigotes found in macrophages of skin and mucous membranes; presence of intracellular forms containing nucleus and kinetoplast diagnostic
Leishmania donovani (visceral)	Amastigotes found throughout reticuloendothelial system and in spleen, liver, bone marrow, etc.; presence of intracellular forms containing nucleus and kinetoplast diagnostic
Wuchereria bancrofti	Microfilariae sheathed, clear space at end of tail; nocturnal periodicity seen; elephantiasis seen in chronic infections
Brugia malayi	Microfilariae sheathed, subterminal and terminal nuclei at end of tail; nocturnal periodicity seen; elephantiasis seen in chronic infections
Loa loa (African eye worm)	Microfilariae sheathed, nuclei continuous to tip of tail; diurnal periodicity; adult worm may cross conjunctiva of eye
Mansonella spp.	Microfilariae unsheathed, nuclei may or may not extend to tip of tail (depending on species); nonperiodic; symptoms usually absent or mild
Mansonella streptocerca	Microfilariae unsheathed, nuclei extend to tip of tail; when immobile, curved like shepherd's crook; adults in dermal tissues
Onchocerca volvulus	Microfilariae unsheathed, nuclei do not extend to tip of tail; adults in nodules

[a]GI, gastrointestinal; RBCs, erythrocytes.
Source: L. S. Garcia and D. A. Bruckner, *Diagnostic Medical Parasitology,* 3rd ed., American Society for Microbiology, Washington, D.C., 1997.

Microbial Identification

Microbial Identification

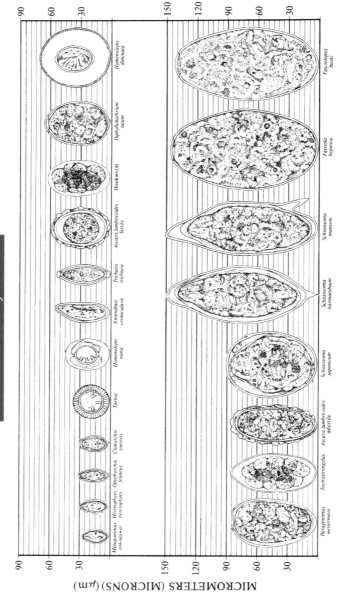

Figure 5.4 Relative sizes of helminth eggs (from Centers for Disease Control and Prevention). *Schistosoma mekongi* and *Schistosoma intercalatum* have been omitted. From M. Brooke and D. Melvin, *Morphology of Diagnostic Stages of Intestinal Parasites of Humans*, 2nd ed., U.S. Department of Health and Human Services publication no. (CDC) 84-8116, Centers for Disease Control and Prevention, Atlanta, Ga., 1984.

Microbial Identification

Table 5.41 Morphological characteristics of helminths

Helminth	Diagnostic stage
Nematodes (roundworms)	
Ascaris lumbricoides	Egg: both fertilized (oval to round with thick, mammillated or tuberculate shell) and unfertilized (tend to be more oval or elongate, with bumpy shell exaggerated) eggs found in stool. Adult worms: 10–12 in. (ca. 25–30 cm), found in stool. Rarely (in severe infections), migrating larvae can be found in sputum.
Trichuris trichiura	Egg: barrel shaped with two clear, polar plugs. Adult worm: rarely seen. Eggs should be quantitated (rare, few, etc.), since light infections may not be treated.
Enterobius vermicularis	Egg: football shaped with one flattened side. Adult worm: about 3/8 in. (ca. 1 cm) long, white with pointed tail. Female migrates from anus and deposits eggs on perianal skin.
Ancylostoma duodenale, Necator americanus	Egg: eggs of two species identical; oval with broadly rounded ends, thin shell, and clear space between shell and developing embryo (8–16-cell stage). Adult worms: rarely seen in clinical specimens.
Strongyloides stercoralis	Rhabditiform larvae (noninfective) usually found in stool; short buccal cavity or capsule with large, genital primordial packet of cells ("short and sexy"). In very heavy infections, larvae are occasionally found in sputum and/or filariform (infective) larvae can be found in stool (slit in tail).
Ancylostoma braziliensis	Humans are accidental hosts. Larvae will wander through outer layer of skin, creating tracks (severe itching and eosinophilia). There are no practical microbiological diagnostic tests.
Toxocara cati or *Toxocara canis*	Humans are accidental hosts. Dog or cat ascarid eggs are ingested with contaminated soil; larvae wander through deep tissues (including eye); can be mistaken for cancer of eye; serologic tests helpful for confirmation; eosinophilia

Cestodes (tapeworms)

Taenia saginata
Scolex (4 suckers, no hooklets) and gravid proglottid (>12 branches on single side) are diagnostic; eggs indicate *Taenia* spp. only (thick, striated shell, containing 6-hooked embryo or oncosphere); worm usually approx 12 ft (ca. 3.7 m) long

Taenia solium
Scolex (4 suckers with hooklets) and gravid proglottid (<12 branches on single side) are diagnostic; eggs indicate *Taenia* spp. only (thick, striated shell, containing 6-hooked embryo or oncosphere); worm usually approx 12 ft (ca. 3.7 m) long

Diphyllobothrium latum
Scolex (lateral sucking grooves) and gravid proglottid (wider than long, reproductive structures in center, "rosette"); eggs operculated

Hymenolepis nana
Adult worm not normally seen; egg round to oval with thin shell, containing 6-hooked embryo or oncosphere with polar filaments lying between embryo and egg shell

Hymenolepis diminuta
Adult worm not normally seen; egg round to oval with thin shell, containing 6-hooked embryo or oncosphere with no polar filaments lying between embryo and egg shell

Echinococcus granulosus
Adult worm found only in carnivores (dog); hydatid cysts develop (primarily in liver) when humans accidentally ingest eggs from dog tapeworms; cyst contains daughter cysts and many scolices. Laboratory should examine fluid aspirated from cyst at surgery.

Echinococcus multilocularis
Adult worm found only in carnivores (fox or wolf); hydatid cysts develop (primarily in liver) when humans accidentally ingest eggs from carnivore tapeworms. Cyst grows like metastatic cancer with no limiting membrane.

(continued)

Microbial Identification

Table 5.41 Morphological characteristics of helminths (*continued*)

Helminth	Diagnostic stage
Trematodes (flukes)	
Fasciolopsis buski	Eggs found in stool; very large and operculated (morphology like that of *Fasciola hepatica* eggs)
Fasciola hepatica	Eggs found in stool; cannot be differentiated from those of *F. buski*
Clonorchis (Opisthorchis) sinensis	Eggs found in stool; very small (<35 μm); operculated, with shoulders into which operculum fits
Paragonimus westermani	Eggs coughed up in sputum (brownish "iron filings" = egg packets); can be recovered in sputum or stool (if swallowed); eggs operculated, with shoulders into which operculum fits
Schistosoma mansoni	Eggs recovered in stool (large lateral spine); specimens should be collected with no preservatives (to maintain egg viability); worms in veins of large intestine
Schistosoma haematobium	Eggs recovered in urine (large terminal spine); specimens should be collected with no preservatives (to maintain egg viability); worms in veins of bladder
Schistosoma japonicum	Eggs recovered in stool (very small lateral spine); specimens should be collected with no preservatives (to maintain egg viability); worms in veins of small intestine

Source: L. S. Garcia and D. A. Bruckner, *Diagnostic Medical Parasitology*, 3rd ed., American Society for Microbiology, Washington, D.C., 1997.

Table 5.42 Key to adult stages of common arthropods of medical importance

---

1. Three or four pairs of legs [2]
   Five or more pairs of legs [22]

2. Three pairs of legs with antennae **(insects: class Insecta)** [3]
   Four pairs of legs without antennae **(spiders, ticks, mites, scorpions: class Arachnida)** [20]

3. Wings present, well developed [4]
   Wings absent or rudimentary [12]

4. One pair of wings **(flies, mosquitos, midges: order Diptera)** [5]
   Two pairs of wings [6]

5. Wings with scales **(mosquitos: order Diptera)**
   Wings without scales **(other flies: order Diptera)**

6. Mouthparts adapted for sucking, with elongate proboscis [7]
   Mouthparts adapted for chewing, without elongate proboscis [8]

7. Wings densely covered with scales, proboscis coiled **(butterflies and moths: order Lepidoptera)**
   Wings not covered with scales; proboscis not coiled but directed backward **(bedbugs and kissing bugs: Hemiptera)**

8. Both pairs of wings membranous, with similar structure, although size may vary [9]
   Front pair of wings leathery or shell-like, serving as covers for second pair [10]

9. Two pairs of wings similar in size **(termites: order Isoptera)**
   Hind wing much smaller than front wing **(wasps, hornets, and bees: order Hymenoptera)**

10. Front wings horny or leathery without distinct veins, meeting in a straight line down the middle [11]
    Front wings leathery or paperlike with distinct veins, usually overlapping in the middle **(cockroaches: order Dictyoptera)**

11. Abdomen with prominent cerci or forceps; wings shorter than abdomen **(earwigs: order Dermaptera)**
    Abdomen without prominent cerci or forceps; wings covering abdomen **(beetles: order Coleoptera)**

12. Abdomen with three long terminal tails **(silverfish and firebrats: order Thysanura)**
    Abdomen without three long terminal tails [13]

13. Abdomen with narrow waist **(ants: order Hymenoptera)**
    Abdomen without narrow waist [14]

14. Abdomen with prominent pair of cerci or forceps **(earwigs: order Dermaptera)**
    Abdomen without cerci or forceps [15]

15. Body flattened laterally; antennae small, fitting into grooves in side of head **(fleas: order Siphonaptera)**
    Body flattened dorsoventrally; antennae projecting from side of head, not fitting into grooves [16]

Microbial Identification

(continued)

Table 5.42 Key to adult stages of common arthropods of medical importance *(continued)*

16. Antennae with nine or more segments [17]
    Antennae with three to five segments [18]

17. Pronotum covering head **(cockroaches: order Dictyoptera)**
    Pronotum not covering head **(termites: order Isoptera)**

18. Mouthparts consisting of tubular jointed beak; three- to
    five-segment tarsi **(bedbugs: order Hemiptera)**
    Mouthparts retracted into head or of chewing type; one- or
    two-segment tarsi [19]

19. Mouthparts retracted into head, adapted for sucking blood
    (sucking lice: order Anopleura)
    Mouthparts of chewing type **(chewing lice: order Mallophaga)**

20. Body oval, consisting of single saclike region **(ticks and mites:
    subclass Acari)**
    Body divided into two distinct regions, a cephalothorax and an
    abdomen [21]

21. Abdomen joined to cephalothorax by slender waist; abdomen
    with segmentation indistinct or absent; stinger absent **(spiders:
    subclass Araneae)**
    Abdomen broadly joined to cephalothorax; abdomen distinctly
    segmented, ending with stinger **(scorpions: subclass Scorpiones)**

22. Five to nine pairs of legs or swimmerets; one or two pairs of
    antennae; principally aquatic organisms **(copepods, crabs, and
    crayfish: class Crustacea)**
    Ten or more pairs of legs; swimmerets absent; one pair of
    antennae; terrestrial organisms [23]

23. Only one pair of legs per body segment **(centipedes: class
    Chilopoda)**
    Two pairs of legs per body segment **(millipedes: class Diplopoda)**

Sources: J. Goddard, *Physician's Guide to Arthropods of Medical Importance*, CRC Press, Inc., Boca Raton, Fla., 1993, and National Communicable Disease Center, *Pictorial Keys: Arthropods, Reptiles, Birds, and Mammals of Public Health Significance*, Communicable Disease Center, Atlanta, Ga., 1969.

Microbial Identification

Vaccines, Antibiotics, and Susceptibility Testing

Infectious diseases can be controlled by two general approaches: immunization and antibiotic therapy. Immunization can be performed with either a live or an inactivated vaccine. The immunization schedule recommended for children and adults in the United States is summarized in the first table of this section.

The determination of antimicrobial susceptibility results for a microbe forms the basis of specific, directed therapy for an active infection. Additionally, the knowledge of susceptibility patterns for groups of organisms is used to guide empiric therapy. It would be impossible to review all testing methods that are currently available or the results of the numerous studies that have characterized susceptibility patterns for all bacteria, viruses, fungi, and parasites. For detailed information about the specifics of susceptibility tests, the reader is referred to the relevant NCCLS documents listed in this section, the *Manual of Clinical Microbiology* (6th ed., 1995), and the *Clinical Microbiology Procedures Handbook* (1992). The information regarding susceptibility patterns has been summarized from numerous scientific publications, data provided by pharmaceutical companies, and national and international studies coordinated by regional reference centers (e.g., the Anti-infective Research Center at the University of Iowa; MRL Pharmaceutical Services in Reston, Va.; the Clinical Microbiology Institute in Tualatin, Oreg.). The data summarized in this section represent national trends. Because susceptibility patterns can vary from one region to another, as well as over time, it is important for each laboratory to determine the relevant antimicrobial susceptibility pattern for the patient population that it serves.

Immunization Recommendations for the United States

Routine Vaccinations

Diphtheria toxoid/tetanus toxoid/acellular pertussis vaccine. Primary vaccination is administered in four doses given at 2, 4, and 6 months and 4–6 years. A booster vaccination with diphtheria and tetanus toxoids is given at 11–12 years. Additional booster vaccination with tetanus toxoid is recommended every 10 years.

Vaccines and Antibiotics

***Haemophilus influenzae* type b (inactivated) vaccine.** Polysaccharide-protein conjugated vaccine is recommended for children and administered in three doses at 2, 4, and 6 months.

Hepatitis B (inactivated) vaccine. This recombinant vaccine is administered in three doses given at birth and 1 and 6 months.

Influenza (inactivated) vaccine. Annual vaccination is recommended for the following: (i) persons ≥65 years; (ii) residents of chronic-care facilities; (iii) adults and children with chronic pulmonary or cardiovascular disorders; (iv) adults and children with chronic metabolic diseases, renal dysfunction, hemoglobinopathies, or immunosuppression; (v) children and teenagers receiving long-term aspirin therapy (at risk of developing Reye's syndrome); and (vi) persons in close contact with high-risk patients (e.g., physicians, nurses, other personnel in hospitals or chronic-care facilities, providers of home care, household members).

Measles/mumps/rubella (live) vaccine. Vaccination is recommended at 12–15 months, with a booster administered at either 4–6 years or 11–12 years.

Pneumococcal (inactivated) vaccine. Vaccination is recommended for the following: (i) immunocompetent persons ≥65 years; (ii) immunocompetent persons 2–64 years with chronic cardiovascular disease, chronic pulmonary disease, diabetes mellitus, alcoholism, chronic liver disease, cerebrospinal fluid leaks, and functional or anatomic asplenia; and (iii) immunocompromised persons aged ≥2 years. This last group should be revaccinated after 5 years (3 years for patients ≤10 years old).

Poliovirus (inactivated and live) vaccines. Three schedules can be used with the inactivated poliovirus vaccine (IPV) and/or the oral poliovirus vaccine (OPV), as follows: (i) administer IPV at 2 and 4 months followed by OPV at 12–18 months and 4–6 years; (ii) administer four doses of IPV at 2 months, 4 months, 12–18 months, and 4–6 years; or (iii) administer four doses of OPV at 2 months, 4 months, 6–18 months, and 4–6 years.

Varicella (live) vaccine. Vaccination is recommended at 12–18 months. Booster vaccination is generally not necessary.

Vaccines and Antibiotics

Special Vaccinations

Adenovirus (live) vaccine. This vaccine was developed against serogroups 4 and 7 and is approved only for use in the military population.

Anthrax (inactivated) vaccine. Vaccination is recommended only for laboratory personnel in contact with *Bacillus anthracis* or individuals who are in contact with imported animal hides, furs, bonemeal, wool, animal hair, and bristles. Vaccination consists of six doses with the first three at 2-week intervals and the remainder at 6-month intervals. Booster doses are recommended at 1-year intervals.

Meningococcal disease (inactivated) vaccine. Vaccine has been developed against serogroups A, C, Y, and W135. Vaccination is recommended for travelers to areas with epidemic meningococcal disease and for individuals with terminal complement component deficiencies or with anatomic or functional asplenia. There is no proven efficacy for booster doses after a single dose.

Plague (inactivated) vaccine. This vaccine is used for sporadic, epidemic, and epizootic infection in Africa, Asia, and South America. Vaccination is recommended for laboratory and field personnel working with *Yersinia pestis* or potentially infected animals, as well as for travelers to rural areas of endemic infection. Primary vaccination consists of three doses administered at 0, 1, and 6 months. Booster doses should be administered at 1- to 2-year intervals.

Rabies (inactivated) vaccine. Preexposure immunization is recommended for high-risk groups including animal handlers, persons in contact with potentially rabid animals, and persons planning to spend more than 1 month in areas where rabies is a constant threat. Continual risk of exposure requires booster vaccination every 2 years or when antibody titers are inadequate. Postexposure vaccination is recommended for persons in contact with saliva or other potentially infectious material from a rabid animal.

Tuberculosis (live) vaccine. Use of the Bacille Calmette-Guérin (BCG) vaccine in the United States is recommended only for children who are unable to receive isoniazid prophylaxis and who are exposed to persons with active disease or those infected with isoniazid-resistant organisms. Vaccination consists of a single percutaneous dose.

Vaccines and Antibiotics

Typhoid (inactivated and live) vaccines. Vaccination is recommended for individuals traveling to areas of endemic infection, particularly to rural areas where prolonged exposure to potentially contaminated food and water is anticipated. Primary vaccination consists of two doses of the inactivated vaccine administered 4 weeks apart or four doses of the live vaccine administered on alternate days. Booster vaccination with the inactivated vaccine should be given every 3 years, while the primary series with the live vaccine should be administered every 5 years.

Vibrio cholerae **(inactivated) vaccine**. Cholera is endemic in Africa, Asia, and South and Central America. Cholera vaccine is indicated for travelers to countries requiring evidence of cholera vaccination for entry, as well as for high-risk groups in areas of endemic infection with unsanitary conditions. The primary vaccination is two doses 1 week to ≥1 month apart. Booster vaccination may be given every 6 months.

Yellow fever (live) vaccine. This vaccine is recommended for persons traveling to or living in areas of endemic infection (Africa and Central and South America). Booster vaccine administered at 10-year intervals.

References

1. **Centers for Disease Control and Prevention**. 1991. Update on adult immunization. Recommendations of the Immunization Practices Advisory Committee. *Morbid. Mortal. Weekly Rep*. **40** (no. RR-12).
2. **Centers for Disease Control and Prevention.** 1996. Immunization of adolescents. Recommendations of the Advisory Committee on Immunization Practices, the American Academy of Pediatrics, the American Academy of Family Physicians, and the American Medical Association. *Morbid. Mortal. Weekly Rep*. **45** (no. RR-13).
3. **Centers for Disease Control and Prevention.** 1997. Recommended childhood immunization schedule—United States. *Morbid. Mortal. Weekly Rep*. **46**:35–40.
4. **Centers for Disease Control and Prevention.** 1997. Prevention of pneumococcal disease. Recommendations of the Advisory Committee on Immunization Practices. *Morbid. Mortal. Weekly Rep*. **46** (no. RR-8).

Table 6.1 List of common antibiotics: generic and trade names

Generic name	Trade name(s)	Trade name	Generic name(s)
Acyclovir	Zovirax	Abelcet	Amphotericin B-lipid
Albendazole	Zentel	Achromycin	Tetracycline
Amantadine	Symadine, Symmetrel	Aerosporin	Polymyxin B
Amdinocillin	Coactin	Albamycin	Novobiocin
Amikacin	Amikin	Alferon	Interferon
p-Aminosalicylic acid	Paser	Amikin	Amikacin
Amoxicillin	Amoxil, Trimox, Wymox	Amoxil	Amoxicillin
Amoxicillin-clavulanate	Augmentin	Amphotec	Amphotericin B-lipid
Amphotericin B	Fungizone	Ancef	Cefazolin
Amphotericin B/lipid	Abelcet, Amphotec	Ancobon	Flucytosine
Ampicillin	Omnipen, Polycillin,	Anspor	Cephradine
	Totacillin	Antepar	Piperazine
		Antiminth	Pyrantel
Ampicillin-sulbactam	Unasyn	Aralen	Chloroquine
Azithromycin	Zithromax	Atabrine	Quinacrine
Aztreonam	Azactam	Augmentin	Amoxicillin-clavulanate
Bacampicillin	Spectrobid	Azactam	Aztreonam
Bacitracin	Baci-IM, Baciguent	AZT	Zidovudine
Butoconazole	Femstat	Baciguent	Bacitracin
Capreomycin	Capastat		

Generic	Trade
Carbenicillin	Geocillin, Geopen
Cefaclor	Ceclor
Cefadroxil	Duricef, Ultracef
Cefamandole	Mandol
Cefazolin	Ancef, Kefzol, Zolicef
Cefepime	Maxipime
Cefixime	Suprax
Cefmetazole	Zefazone
Cefonicid	Monocid
Cefoperazone	Cefobid
Ceforanide	Precef
Cefotaxime	Claforan
Cefotetan	Cefotan
Cefoxitin	Mefoxin
Cefpodoxime	Vantin
Cefprozil	Cefzil
Ceftazidime	Ceptaz, Fortaz, Tazicef, Tazidime
Ceftibuten	Cedax
Ceftizoxime	Cefizox
Ceftriaxone	Rocephin

Generic	Trade
Bacitracin	Baci-IM
Oxacillin	Bactocill
Trimethoprim-sulfamethoxazole, co-trimoxazole	Bactrim
Mupirocin	Bactroban
Clarithromycin	Biaxin
Penicillin G	Bicillin
Praziquantel	Biltricide
Capreomycin	Capastat
Cefaclor	Ceclor
Ceftibutin	Cedax
Cephapirin	Cefadyl
Cephalexin	Cefanex
Ceftizoxime	Cefizox
Cefoperazone	Cefobid
Cefotetan	Cefotan
Cefuroxime	Ceftin
Cefprozil	Cefzil
Methicillin	Celbenin
Ceftazidime	Ceptaz
Chloramphenicol	Chloromycetin

(continued)

Table 6.1 List of common antibiotics: generic and trade names *(continued)*

Generic name	Trade name(s)	Trade name	Generic name(s)
Cefuroxime	Ceftin, Kefurox, Zinacef	Cinobac	Cinoxacin
Cephalexin	Cefanex, Keflex, Keftab	Cipro	Ciprofloxacin
Cephalothin	Keflin	Claforan	Cefotaxime
Cephapirin	Cefadyl	Cleocin	Clindamycin
Cephradine	Anspor, Velocef	Cloxapen	Cloxacillin
Chloramphenicol	Chloromycetin	Coactin	Amdinocillin
Chloroquine	Aralen, Plaquenil	Coly-Mycin M	Colistin
Cidofovir	Vistide	Cotrim	Trimethoprim-sulfamethoxazole, co-trimoxazole
Cinoxacin	Cinobac		
Ciprofloxacin	Cipro		
Clarithromycin	Biaxin	Crixivan	Indinavir
Clindamycin	Cleocin	Cytovene	Ganciclovir
Clofazimine	Lamprene	Dapsone	Dapsone
Clotrimazole	Lotrimin, Mycelex	Daraprim	Pyrimethamine
Cloxacillin	Cloxapen, Tegopen	ddC	Zalcitabine
Colistin	Coly-Mycin M	ddI	Didanosine
Co-trimoxazole	Bactrim, Cotrim, Septra, Sulfatrim, Triazole	Dendrid	Idoxuridine
		Diflucan	Fluconazole
Cycloserine	Seromycin	Doryx	Doxycycline

(continued)

Dapsone	Dapsone	Duracillin	Penicillin G
Dicloxacillin	Dynapen, Dycill, Pathocil	Duricef	Cefadroxil
Didanosine	ddI, Videx	Dycill	Dicloxacillin
Diethylcarbamazine	Hetrazan	Dynabac	Dirithromycin
Diloxanide	Furamide	Dynapen	Dicloxacillin
Dirithromycin	Dynabac	Ecostatin	Econazole
Doxycycline	Doryx, Vibramycin	Emetine	Emetine
Econazole	Ecostatin	Epivir	Lamivudine
Emetine	Emetine	Erythrocin	Erythromycin
Enoxacin	Penetrex	Famvir	Famciclovir
Erythromycin	Erythrocin, Pediamycin	Fansidar	Sulfadoxine-pyrimethamine
Erythromycin-sulfisoxazole	Pediazole, Sulfamycin	Femstat	Butoconazole
Ethambutol	Myambutol	Flagyl	Metronidazole
Ethionamide	Trecator	Floxin	Ofloxacin
Famciclovir	Famvir	Flumadine	Rimantadine
Fluconazole	Diflucan	Fortaz	Ceftazidime
Flucytosine	Ancobon	Foscavir	Foscarnet
Foscarnet	Foscavir	Fulvicin	Griseofulvin
Furazolidone	Furoxone	Fungizone	Amphotericin B
Ganciclovir	Cytovene	Furacin	Nitrofurazone
Gentamicin	Garamycin, Jenamicin	Furadantin	Nitrofurantoin

Vaccines and Antibiotics

Vaccines and Antibiotics

Table 6.1 List of common antibiotics: generic and trade names *(continued)*

Generic name	Trade name(s)	Trade name	Generic name(s)
Griseofulvin	Fulvicin, Grifulvin, Grisactin	Furamide	Diloxanide
		Furoxone	Furazolidone
Idoxuridine	Dendrid, Stoxil	Gantrisin	Sulfisoxazole
Imipenem-cilastatin	Primaxin	Garamycin	Gentamicin
Indinavir	Crixivan	Geocillin	Carbenicillin
Interferon	Alferon, Roferon-A	Geopen	Carbenicillin
Iodoquinol	Yodoxin	Gramicidin	Polymyxin B
Isoniazid	Nydrazid, Tubizid	Grifulvin	Griseofulvin
Itraconazole	Sporanox	Grisactin	Griseofulvin
Ivermectin	Mectizan	Hetrazan	Diethylcarbamazine
Kanamycin	Kantrex	Hiprex	Methenamine
Ketoconazole	Nizoral	Hivid	Zalcitabine
Lamivudine	Epivir	Humatin	Paromomycin
Levofloxacin	Levoquin	Invirase	Saquinavir
Leucovorin	Wellcovorin	Jenamicin	Gentamicin
Lincomycin	Lincocin	Kantrex	Kanamycin
Lindane	Kwell	Keflex	Cephalexin
Lomefloxacin	Maxaquin	Keflin	Cephalothin
Loracarbef	Lorabid	Keftab	Cephalexin

(continued)

Generic	Brand
Mebendazole	Vermox
Mefloquine	Lariam
Meparcrine	Quinacrine
Meropenem	Merrem
Methacycline	Rondomycin
Methenamine	Hiprex, Mandelamine, Urex
Methicillin	Celbenin, Staphcillin
Metronidazole	Flagyl, Protostat
Mezlocillin	Mezlin
Miconazole	Monistat
Minocycline	Minocin
Mupirocin	Bactroban
Nafcillin	Nafcil, Unipen
Nalidixic acid	NegGram
Nelfinavir	Viracept
Neomycin	Mycifradin
Netilmicin	Netromycin
Nevirapine	Viramune
Niclosamide	Niclocide
Nitrofurantoin	Furadantin, Macrobid, Macrodantin

Brand	Generic
Kefurox	Cefuroxime
Kefzol	Cefazolin
Kwell	Lindane
Lamisil	Terbinafine
Lamprene	Clofazimine
Lariam	Mefloquine
Levoquin	Levofloxacin
Lincocin	Lincomycin
Lorabid	Loracarbef
Lotrimin	Clotrimazole
Lyphocin	Vancomycin
Macrobid	Nitrofurantoin
Macrodantin	Nitrofurantoin
Mandelamine	Methenamine
Mandol	Cefamandole
Maxaquin	Lomefloxacin
Maxipime	Cefepime
Mectizan	Ivermectin
Mefoxin	Cefoxitin
Merrem	Meropenem
Mezlin	Mezlocillin

Vaccines and Antibiotics

Table 6.1 List of common antibiotics: generic and trade names *(continued)*

Generic name	Trade name(s)	Trade name	Generic name(s)
Nitrofurazone	Furacin	Minocin	Minocycline
Norfloxacin	Noroxin	Mintezol	Thiabendazole
Novobiocin	Albamycin	Monistat	Miconazole
Nystatin	Mycostatin, Nystex, Nilstat	Monocid	Cefonicid
Ofloxacin	Floxin	Myambutol	Ethambutol
Oxacillin	Bactocill, Prostaphlin	Mycelex	Clotrimazole
Oxytetracycline	Terramycin	Mycifradin	Neomycin
Paromomyin	Humatin	Mycobutin	Rifabutin
Pefloxacin	Peflacine	Mycostatin	Nystatin
Penicillin G	Bicillin, Duracillin, Permapen	Nafcil	Nafcillin
		Nebcin	Tobramycin
Penicillin V	Pen-Vee	NebuPent	Pentamidine
Pentamidine	NebuPent, Pentam	NegGram	Nalidixic acid
Piperacillin	Pipracil	Netromycin	Netilmicin
Piperacillin-tazobactam	Zosyn	Niclocide	Niclosamide
Piperazine	Antepar	Nilstat	Nystatin
Polymyxin B	Aerosporin, Gramicidin	Nizoral	Ketoconazole
Praziquantel	Biltricide	Noroxin	Norfloxacin
Primaquine	Primaquine	Norvir	Ritonavir

(continued)

Pyrantel	Antiminth	Nydrazid	Isoniazid
Pyrazinamide	Pyrazinamide	Nystex	Nystatin
Pyrimethamine	Daraprim	Omnipen	Ampicillin
Quinacrine	Atabrine	Pathocil	Dicloxacillin
Quinine	Quinamm, Quindan,	Paser	p-Aminosalicylic acid
	Quiphile	Pediamycin	Erythromycin
Quinupristin-dalfopristin	Synercid	Pediazole	Erythromycin-sulfisoxazole
Ribavirin	Virazole	Peflacine	Pefloxacin
Rifabutin	Mycobutin	Penetrex	Enoxacin
Rifampin	Rifadin, Rifamate, Rifater,	Pentam	Pentamidine
	Rimactane	Pen-Vee	Penicillin V
Rimantadine	Flumadine	Permapen	Penicillin G
Ritonavir	Norvir	Pipracil	Piperacillin
Saquinavir	Invirase	Plaquenil	Chloroquine
Somatropin	Serostim	Polycillin	Ampicillin
Sparfloxacin	Zagam	Precef	Ceforanide
Spectinomycin	Trobicin	Primaquine	Primaquine
Stavudine	Zerit	Primaxin	Imipenem-cilastatin
Streptomycin	Streptomycin	Proloprim	Trimethoprim
Sulfadoxine-pyrimethamine	Fansidar	Prostaphlin	Oxacillin
Sulfisoxazole	Gantrisin	Protostat	Metronidazole

Vaccines and Antibiotics

Vaccines and Antibiotics

Table 6.1 List of common antibiotics: generic and trade names *(continued)*

Generic name	Trade name(s)	Trade name	Generic name(s)
Terbinafine	Lamisil	Pyrazinamide	Pyrazinamide
Tetracycline	Achromycin	Quinacrine	Mepacrine
Thiabendazole	Mintezol	Quinamm	Quinine
Ticarcillin	Ticar	Quindan	Quinine
Ticarcillin-clavulanate	Timentin	Quiphile	Quinine
Tobramycin	Nebcin, Tobrex	Retrovir	Zidovudine
Trifluridine	Viroptic	Rifadin	Rifampin
Trimethoprim	Proloprim, Trimpex	Rifamate	Rifampin
Trimethoprim-sulfamethoxazole	Bactrim, Cotrim, Septra,	Rifater	Rifampin
	Sulfatrim, Triazole	Rimactane	Rifampin
Vancomycin	Lyphocin, Vancocin,	Rocephin	Ceftriaxone
	Vancor	Roferon-A	Interferon
Valacyclovir	Valtrex	Rondomycin	Methacycline
Zalcitabine	ddC, Hivid	Septra	Trimethoprim-sulfamethoxazole,
Zidovudine	AZT, Retrovir		co-trimoxazole
		Seromycin	Cycloserine
		Serostim	Somatropin
		Spectrobid	Bacampicillin
		Sporanox	Itraconazole

Staphcillin	Methicillin
Stoxil	Idoxuridine
Streptomycin	Streptomycin
Sulfamycin	Erythromycin-sulfisoxazole
Sulfatrim	Trimethoprim-sulfamethoxazole, co-trimoxazole
Suprax	Cefixime
Symadine	Amantadine
Symmetrel	Amantadine
Synercid	Quinupristin-dalfopristin
Tazicef	Ceftazidime
Tazidime	Ceftazidime
Tegopen	Cloxacillin
Terramycin	Oxytetracycline
Ticar	Ticarcillin
Timentin	Ticarcillin-clavulanic acid
Tobrex	Tobramycin
Totacillin	Ampicillin
Trecator	Ethionamide
Triazole	Trimethoprim-sulfamethoxazole, co-trimoxazole

(continued)

Vaccines and Antibiotics

Table 6.1 List of common antibiotics: generic and trade names *(continued)*

Generic name	Trade name(s)	Trade name	Generic name(s)
		Trimox	Amoxicillin
		Trimpex	Trimethoprim
		Trobicin	Spectinomycin
		Tubizid	Isoniazid
		Uracef	Cefadroxil
		Unasyn	Ampicillin-sulbactam
		Unipen	Nafcillin
		Urex	Methenamine
		Valtrex	Valacyclovir
		Vancocin	Vancomycin
		Vancor	Vancomycin
		Vantin	Cefpodoxime
		Velocef	Cephradine
		Vermox	Mebendazole
		Vibramycin	Doxycycline
		Videx	Didanosine
		Viracept	Nelfinavir
		Viramune	Nevirapine
		Virazole	Ribavirin

Viroptic	Trifluridine
Vistide	Cidofovir
Wellcovorin	Leucovorin
Wymox	Amoxicillin
Yodoxin	Iodoquinol
Zagam	Sparfloxacin
Zefazone	Cefmetazole
Zentel	Albendazole
Zerit	Stavudine
Zinacef	Cefuroxime
Zithromax	Azithromycin
Zolicef	Cefazolin
Zosyn	Piperacillin-tazobactam
Zovirax	Acyclovir

Vaccines and Antibiotics

Table 6.2 Pharmacokinetic properties of antibacterial, antiviral, antifungal, and antiparasitic agents[a]

Antimicrobial agent	Unit dose	Avg peak level in serum (μg/ml)[b]		
		p.o.	i.m.	i.v.
Acyclovir	200 mg	0.6		
	5 mg/kg			8.8
Albendazole	15 mg/kg	0.8		
Amantadine	200 mg	0.2–0.9		
Amikacin	7.5 mg/kg		15–20	20–40
p-Aminosalicylic acid	4 g	7–8		
Amoxicillin	500 mg	6–8		
Amoxicillin-clavulanate	500/125 mg	4.4 (amox)		
		2.3 (clav)		
Amphotericin B	0.65 mg/kg	1.8–3.5		
Ampicillin	500 mg	2.5–5	8–10	
	1 g			40
Ampicillin-sulbactam	3 g			120 (amp)
				60 (sulb)
	1.5 g		18 (amp)	
			13 (sulb)	
Azithromycin	500 mg	0.4		3.6
Aztreonam	1 g		45	90–160

	Dose			
Capreomycin	1 g		30–35	
Carbenicillin	1 g		20–30	150
Carbenicillin indanyl sodium	764 mg	10		
Cefaclor	500 mg	16		
Cefadroxil	500 mg	10		
Cefamandole	1 g		20–36	90–140
Cefazolin	1 g		65	185
Cefepime	1 g		30	65
Cefixime	400 mg	3.5		
Cefmetazole	1 g			70
Cefonicid	1 g		98	220
Cefoperazone	1 g		65–75	153
Ceforanide	1 g		70	125
Cefotaxime	1 g		20	40–45
Cefotetan	1 g		50–80	160
Cefoxitin	1 g		20–25	55–110
Cefpirome	1 g		45	86
Cefpodoxime	200 mg	2.3		
Cefprozil	500 mg	10.5		70
Ceftazidime	1 g		40	
Ceftizoxime	1 g		39	80–90

(continued)

Vaccines and Antibiotics

Table 6.2 Pharmacokinetic properties of antibacterial, antiviral, antifungal, and antiparasitic agents[a] *(continued)*

Antimicrobial agent	Unit dose	Avg peak level in serum (μg/ml)[b]		
		p.o.	i.m.	i.v.
Ceftriaxone	500 mg		40–45	
	1 g			150
Cefuroxime	750 mg		27	50
Cefuroxime axetil	500 mg	9		
Cephalexin	500 mg	18		
Cephalothin	1 g			30–60
Cephapirin	1 g			40–70
Cephradine	500 mg	16		
	1 g		12	60–80
Chloramphenicol	1 g	10–18		10–15
Cinoxacin	500 mg	15		
Ciprofloxacin	500 mg	2.5		
	400 mg			4.6
Clarithromycin	250 mg	0.5–1		
Clindamycin	300 mg	3	6	
	600 mg			10–12
Clotrimazole	20 mg/kg	0.5–1.5		
Cloxacillin	500 mg	10		

Colistimethate sodium	150 mg		5–6	
Cycloserine	250 mg	10		
Didanosine	300 mg	1.6		
Dirithromycin	500 mg	0.45		
Dicloxacillin	500 mg	15		
Doxycycline	100 mg	2.5		
Enoxacin	400 mg	3–5		
Erythromycin	500 mg	2–3		4
	1 g			10
Ethambutol	25 mg/kg	5		
Ethionamide	250 mg	2		
Famciclovir	500 mg	3–4		
Fleroxacin	400 mg	5		7–8
Fluconazole	400 mg/kg	4.1–8.0		
5-Flucytosine	2 g	45		50
Foscarnet	57 mg/kg			575 µmol/liter
Fusidic acid	500 mg	25–30		50
Ganciclovir	5 mg/kg			8.3
Gentamicin	1.5 mg/kg		4–6	4–8
Griseofulvin	1 g	1–2		
Imipenem	500 mg			25–35

(continued)

Vaccines and Antibiotics

Vaccines and Antibiotics

Table 6.2 Pharmacokinetic properties of antibacterial, antiviral, antifungal, and antiparasitic agents[a] *(continued)*

Antimicrobial agent	Unit dose	Avg peak level in serum (μg/ml)[b]		
		p.o.	i.m.	i.v.
Isoniazid	300 mg	7		
	800 mg	10–15		
Itraconazole	200 mg	1.1–2.3		
Kanamycin	7.5 mg/kg		20–25	
Ketoconazole	200 mg	3–4.5		
	400 mg	7		
Lomefloxacin	500 mg	5.7		6.4
Loracarbef	400 mg	14		
Mefloquine	250 mg	0.3		
	1 g	0.5–1.2		
Meropenem	500 mg			25–35
Metronidazole	500 mg	12		20–25
Mezlocillin	1 g		15	
	3 g			260
Miconazole	200 mg	0.1		1.6
	1 g	0.5–1		
Minocycline	100 mg	1		
Nafcillin	500 mg		5–8	

Antibiotic	Dose			
Nalidixic acid	1 g	20–50		20–40
Netilmicin	2 mg/kg		5–7	6–8
Nitrofurantoin	100 mg	<2		
Norfloxacin	400 mg	1.5		
Ofloxacin	400 mg	4		
Oxacillin	500 mg	4–6		
	1 g		14–16	40
Oxytetracycline	250 mg	3–4		
Pefloxacin	400 mg	3		
Penicillin G	500 mg	1.5–2.5		
Aqueous	1×10^6 U		8–10	10
Benzathine	1.2×10^6 U		0.1–0.15	
Procaine	1.2×10^6 U		3	
Penicillin V	500 mg	3–5		
Pentamidine	4 mg/kg		36	0.5–3.4
Piperacillin	2 g			240
	4 g			
Piperacillin-tazobactam	2.25 g		38 (pip)	280 (pip)
	4.5 g		7 (tazo)	

(continued)

Vacines and Antibiotics

Table 6.2 Pharmacokinetic properties of antibacterial, antiviral, antifungal, and antiparasitic agents[a] *(continued)*

Antimicrobial agent	Unit dose	Avg peak level in serum (µg/ml)[b]		
		p.o.	i.m.	i.v.
Polymyxin B	2.5 mg/kg			35 (tazo)
Pyrazinamide	0.5 g	5		5
	3 g	30		
Pyrimethamine	25 mg	0.1–0.3		
Quinine	650 mg	3–10		
Ribavirin	1 g	1–3		
Rifampin	600 mg	7–9		10
Rimantadine	200 mg	0.4		
Sparfloxacin	200 mg	2.3		
Spectinomycin	2 g			100
Spiramycin	2 g	3		
Stavudine	70 mg	1.4		
Streptomycin	1 g		25–50	
Sulfadiazine	2 g	100–150		
Sulfadoxine	1 g	50–75		
Sulfamethizole	2 g	60		
Sulfamethoxazole	1 g	40		

	Dose			
Sulfisoxazole	2 g	170		
Teicoplanin	200 mg		7	20–40
Tetracycline	400 mg	4		
	500 mg			8
Ticarcillin	1 g		20–30	
	3 g			190
Ticarcillin-clavulanate	3.1 g			330 (ticar)
				8 (clav)
Tobramycin	1.5 mg/kg		4–6	4–8
Trimethoprim	100 mg	1		
Trimethoprim-sulfamethoxazole	160/800 mg	3 (TMP)		9 (TMP)
		46 (SMX)		106 (SMX)
Trovafloxacin	200 mg	3.1		3.1
Vancomycin	500 mg			20–40
Zalcitabine	0.5 mg	7.6 ng/ml		
Zidovudine	200 mg	1.1		

[a] Table adapted from P. R. Murray, E. J Baron, M. A. Pfaller, F. C. Tenover, and R. H. Yolken (ed.), *Manual of Clinical Microbiology*, 6th ed., ASM Press, Washington, D.C., 1995 (p. 1300), and A. Kucers and N. M. Bennet, *The Use of Antibiotics*, 4th ed., J. B. Lippincott Co., Philadelphia, 1989.

[b] p.o., administered orally; i.m., administered intramuscularly; i.v., administered intravenously.

Vaccines and Antibiotics

Table 6.3 National Committee for Clinical Laboratory
Standards (NCCLS) documents related to antimicrobial
susceptibility testing[a]

No.	Title
M2-A6	Performance Standards for Antimicrobial Disk Susceptibility Tests (1997)
M6-A	Protocols for Evaluating Dehydrated Mueller-Hinton Agar (1996)
M7-A4	Methods for Dilution Antimicrobial Susceptibility Tests for Bacteria That Grow Aerobically (1997)
M11-A4	Methods for Antimicrobial Susceptibility Testing of Anaerobic Bacteria (1997)
M21-T	Methodology for the Serum Bactericidal Test (1992)
M23-A	Development of In Vitro Susceptibility Testing Criteria and Quality Control Parameters (1994)
M24-T	Antimycobacterial Susceptibility Testing for *Mycobacterium tuberculosis* (1995)
M26-T	Methods for Determining Bactericidal Activity of Antimicrobial Agents (1992)
M27-A	Reference Method for Broth Dilution Antifungal Susceptibility Testing of Yeasts (1997)
M31-T	Performance Standards for Antimicrobial Disk and Dilution Susceptibility Tests for Bacteria Isolated from Animals (1997)
M33	Antiviral Susceptibility Testing (under development)
M37-P	Development of In Vitro Susceptibility Testing Criteria and Quality Control Parameters for Veterinary Antimicrobial Agents (1996)
M38	Reference Method for Broth Dilution Antifungal Susceptibility Testing of Filamentous Fungi (under development)
M100-S8	Performance Standards for Antimicrobial Susceptibility Testing (1998)
SC21-L	Susceptibility Testing (collection of documents: M2, M7, M11, M21, M24, M27, M31, and M100)

[a]Documents available from NCCLS (940 West Valley Road, Suite 1400, Wayne, PA 19087; telephone, 610-688-0100; FAX, 610-688-0700; E-mail, exofice@nccls.org; Website, http://www.nccls.org).

Table 6.4   Quality control organisms for antimicrobial susceptibility tests

Quality control organism	Test(s)
Staphylococcus aureus ATCC 25923	Disk diffusion and broth dilution
Staphylococcus aureus ATCC 29213	Disk diffusion and broth dilution
Enterococcus faecalis ATCC 29212	Disk diffusion and agar and broth dilution
Enterococcus faecalis ATCC 51299	Agar and broth dilution
Escherichia coli ATCC 25922	Disk diffusion and broth dilution
Escherichia coli ATCC 35218	Disk diffusion and broth dilution
Pseudomonas aeruginosa ATCC 27853	Disk diffusion and broth dilution
Haemophilus influenzae ATCC 49247	Disk diffusion and broth dilution
Haemophilus influenzae ATCC 49766	Disk diffusion and broth dilution
Neisseria gonorrhoeae ATCC 49226	Disk diffusion and broth dilution
Streptococcus pneumoniae ATCC 49619	Disk diffusion and broth dilution
Bacteroides fragilis ATCC 25285	Agar and broth dilution
Bacteroides thetaiotaomicron ATCC 29741	Agar and broth dilution
Eubacterium lentum ATCC 43055	Agar and broth dilution
Nocardia asteroides ATCC 19247	Broth dilution
Mycobacterium tuberculosis (H37Rv) ATCC 27294	Agar dilution and BACTEC
Mycobacterium tuberculosis (H37Rv; streptomycin resistant) ATCC 35820	Agar dilution and BACTEC
Mycobacterium tuberculosis (H37Rv; *p*-aminosalicylic acid resistant) ATCC 35821	Agar dilution and BACTEC
Mycobacterium tuberculosis (H37Rv; isoniazid resistant) ATCC 35822	Agar dilution and BACTEC
Mycobacterium tuberculosis (H37Rv; cycloserine resistant) ATCC 35826	Agar dilution and BACTEC

Vaccines and Antibiotics

(continued)

Table 6.4 Quality control organisms for antimicrobial
susceptibility tests *(continued)*

Quality control organism	Test(s)
Mycobacterium tuberculosis (H37Rv; kanamycin resistant) ATCC 35827	Agar dilution and BACTEC
Mycobacterium tuberculosis (H37Rv; pyrazinamide resistant) ATCC 35828	Agar dilution and BACTEC
Mycobacterium tuberculosis (H37Rv; ethionamide resistant) ATCC 35830	Agar dilution and BACTEC
Mycobacterium tuberculosis (H37Rv; ethambutol resistant) ATCC 35837	Agar dilution and BACTEC
Mycobacterium tuberculosis (H37Rv; rifampin resistant) ATCC 35838	Agar dilution and BACTEC
Mycobacterium fortuitum ATCC 6841	Agar elution and broth dilution
Candida parapsilosis ATCC 22019 (QC strain)	Broth dilution
Candida krusei ATCC 6258 (QC strain)	Broth dilution
Candida parapsilosis ATCC 90018 (reference strain)	Broth dilution
Candida albicans ATCC 90028 (reference strain)	Broth dilution
Candida albicans ATCC 24433 (reference strain)	Broth dilution
Candida tropicalis ATCC 750 (reference strain)	Broth dilution

Vaccines and Antibiotics

Table 6.5 Summary of antimicrobial susceptibility test methods for bacteria, mycobacteria, and fungi[a]

Organism	Test method	Medium	Inoculum	Incubation conditions
Staphylococcus spp.	Disk diffusion	MHA	Direct	Air; 16–18 h (oxac: 24 h); 35°C
	Broth/agar dilution	CAMHB or MHA (oxac + 2% NaCl)	Direct	Air; 16–18 h (oxac: 24 h); 35°C
	Agar screen (oxac)	MHA + 4% NaCl + oxac (6 μg/ml)	Direct	Air; 24 h (CNS: 48 h); 35°C
Streptococcus pneumoniae	Disk diffusion	MHA + 5% sheep blood	Direct	5% CO$_2$; 20–24 h; 35°C
	Broth dilution	CAMHB + 2–5% LHB	Direct	Air; 20–24 h; 35°C
Streptococcus, other spp.	Disk diffusion	MHA + 5% sheep blood	Direct	5% CO$_2$; 20–24 h; 35°C
	Broth/agar dilution	CAMHB + 2–5% LHB, or MHA + 5% sheep blood	Direct	5% CO$_2$ (agar) or air (broth); 20–24 h; 35°C
Enterococcus spp.	Disk diffusion	MHA	Direct; broth	Air; 16–18 h (vanco: 24 h); 35°C
	Broth/agar dilution	CAMHB or MHA	Direct; broth	Air; 16–18 h (vanco: 24 h); 35°C

(continued)

Vaccines and Antibiotics

Vaccines and Antibiotics

Table 6.5 Summary of antimicrobial susceptibility test methods for bacteria, mycobacteria, and fungi[a] *(continued)*

Organism	Test method	Medium	Inoculum	Incubation conditions
	Agar screen	BHIA + gent (500 µg/ml)	Direct; broth	Air; 24 h; 35°C
		BHIA + strep (2,000 µg/ml)	Direct; broth	Air; 24 h; 35°C
		BHIA + vanco (6 µg/ml)	Direct; broth	Air; 24 h; 35°C
Listeria spp.	Broth dilution	CAMHB + 2–5% LHB	Direct; broth	Air; 18 h; 35°C
Neisseria gonorrhoeae	Disk diffusion	GCA + 1% supplement	Direct	5% CO_2; 20–24 h; 35°C
	Agar dilution	GCA + 1% supplement	Direct	5% CO_2; 20–24 h; 35°C
Neisseria meningitidis	Broth/agar dilution	CAMHB + 2–5% LHB	Direct	5% CO_2; 24 h; 35°C
		MHA + 5% sheep blood	Direct	5% CO_2; 24 h; 35°C
Haemophilus spp.	Disk diffusion	HTM agar	Direct	5% CO_2; 16–18 h; 35°C
	Broth dilution	HTM broth	Direct	Air; 20–24 h; 35°C
Enterobacteriaceae	Disk diffusion	MHA	Direct; broth	Air; 16–18 h; 35°C
	Broth/agar dilution	CAMHB or MHA	Direct; broth	Air; 16–20 h; 35°C
Vibrio cholerae	Disk diffusion	MHA	Direct; broth	Air; 16–18 h; 35°C
	Broth/agar dilution	CAMHB or MHA	Direct; broth	Air; 16–20 h; 35°C
Pseudomonas aeruginosa	Disk diffusion	MHA	Direct; broth	Air; 16–20 h; 35°C
	Broth/agar dilution	CAMHB or MHA	Direct; broth	Air; 16–20 h; 35°C

Acinetobacter spp.	Disk diffusion	MHA	Direct; broth	Air; 16–20 h; 35°C
	Broth/agar dilution	CAMHB/MHA	Direct; broth	Air; 16–20 h; 35°C
Pseudomonas, other spp.	Broth/agar dilution	CAMHB or MHA	Direct; broth	Air; 16–20 h; 35°C
Anaerobes	Broth/agar dilution	Brucella broth/agar + hemin (5 μg/ml), vitamin K_1 (1 μg/ml), 5% lysed sheep blood	Direct; broth	Anaerobic; 48 h; 35–37°C
Nocardia spp.	Broth dilution	CAMHB	Direct; broth	Air; 2–5 days; 35°C
Mycobacteria, rapid growers	Broth dilution	CAMHB + 0.02% Tween 80	Direct; broth	Air; 3–5 days; 30°C
	Agar disk elution	MHA + OADC	Direct; broth	Air; 3–5 days; 30°C
Mycobacteria, slow growers	Proportion agar dilution	7H10 agar + OADC	Direct; broth	5–10% CO_2; 3 wks; 37°C
	BACTEC broth	BACTEC 12B broth	Direct; broth	5–10% CO_2; 5–14 days; 37°C
Fungi (yeasts)	Broth dilution	RPMI 1640 broth	Broth	Air; 46–50 h (*Cryptococcus:* 70–74 h); 35°C

[a]Inoculum can be prepared either directly with isolated colonies on an agar plate (direct) or after growth of the organism in a broth culture (broth). Abbreviations: MHA, Mueller-Hinton agar; CAMHB, cation-adjusted Mueller-Hinton broth; NaCl, sodium chloride; LHB, lysed horse blood; BHIA, brain heart infusion agar; GCA, GC agar; HTM, Haemophilus test medium; OADC, oleic acid supplement; CNS, coagulase-negative staphylococci; oxac, oxacillin; gent, gentamicin; strep, streptomycin; vanco, vancomycin.

Vaccines and Antibiotics

Table 6.6 Susceptibility patterns for aerobic gram-positive bacteria

Organism	Generally active[a]	Unpredictable activity	Generally inactive
Enterococcus faecalis	**(Penicillin or ampicillin or vancomycin) + gentamicin**, nitrofurantoin	Quinolones, imipenem	All cephalosporins, oxacillin, TMP-SMX[b], macrolides, clindamycin
Enterococcus faecium		Vancomycin + (gentamicin or streptomycin), quinolones	Penicillin, ampicillin, oxacillin, all cephalosporins, imipenem, TMP-SMX, macrolides, clindamycin
Staphylococcus spp. (oxacillin susceptible)	**Oxacillin, vancomycin,** cephalosporins, imipenem, macrolides, clindamycin, quinolones	Aminoglycosides	Penicillin
Staphylococcus (oxacillin resistant)	**Vancomycin**	Imipenem, quinolones	Penicillin, oxacillin, cephalosporins, macrolides, clindamycin, aminoglycosides
Stomatococcus spp.	**Penicillin,** cephalosporins, imipenem, vancomycin	Aminoglycosides, clindamycin, macrolides	
Streptococcus spp., beta-hemolytic	**Penicillin,** cephalosporins, imipenem, vancomycin	Quinolones, macrolides	Aminoglycosides

Organism			
Streptococcus, viridans group	**Vancomycin or cephalosporins [if penicillin resistant]**, imipenem	**Penicillin [if susceptible]**, quinolones, macrolides	Aminoglycosides
Streptococcus pneumoniae	**Vancomycin or cephalosporins [if penicillin resistant]**, imipenem	**Penicillin [if susceptible]**, quinolones, macrolides	Aminoglycosides, tetracycline
Arcanobacterium haemolyticum	**Penicillin**, cephalosporins, imipenem, vancomycin, macrolides, clindamycin, tetracyclines, quinolones		TMP-SMX
Bacillus anthracis	**Penicillin**, quinolones, macrolides, tetracycline, chloramphenicol		Cephalosporins
Bacillus cereus	**Vancomycin**, imipenem, chloramphenicol, macrolides, clindamycin, quinolones, gentamicin	Sulfonamides, tetracycline	Penicillins, cephalosporins
Corynebacterium diphtheriae	**Penicillin, erythromycin**, cephalosporins, vancomycin, quinolones, aminoglycosides	TMP-SMX	
Corynebacterium jeikeium	**Vancomycin**	Quinolones	Penicillins, cephalosporins, macrolides, clindamycin, aminoglycosides

(continued)

Vaccines and Antibiotics

Table 6.6 Susceptibility patterns for aerobic gram-positive bacteria *(continued)*

Organism	Generally active[a]	Unpredictable activity	Generally inactive
Corynebacterium urealyticum	**Vancomycin**	Quinolones, macrolides, tetracyclines	Penicillins, cephalosporins, aminoglycosides
Erysipelothrix rhusiopathiae	**Penicillin**, cephalosporins, imipenem, macrolides, clindamycin, quinolones, chloramphenicol		Aminoglycosides, TMP-SMX, vancomycin
Leuconostoc spp.	**Imipenem**, chloramphenicol, aminoglycosides, tetracyclines	Penicillins, cephalosporins	Vancomycin
Listeria monocytogenes	**Penicillin [ampicillin] + aminoglycoside**, vancomycin	Quinolones, macrolides, clindamycin, TMP-SMX	Cephalosporins
Nocardia farcinica	**Sulfonamides**, amikacin	Imipenem, quinolones	Penicillins, cephalosporins, macrolides
Nocardia, other spp.	**Sulfonamides**, imipenem, amikacin	Quinolones, cephalosporins [broad-spectrum]	Penicillins, macrolides
Rhodococcus equi	**Vancomycin**, aminoglycosides, quinolones	Macrolides, clindamycin, tetracyclines	Penicillins, cephalosporins, TMP-SMX
Tsukamurella paurometabolum	**Imipenem**, aminoglycosides, quinolones	TMP-SMX, tetracyclines	Penicillins, cephalosporins, macrolides

[a]Therapy of choice in bold type. Parentheses indicate alternative choices. Brackets indicate specific details.
[b]TMP-SMX, trimethoprim-sulfamethoxazole.

Table 6.7 Susceptibility of common gram-negative bacilli to selected penicillins

Organism	MIC$_{90}$/% susceptible			
	Ampicillin-sulbactam	Ticarcillin-clavulanate	Piperacillin-tazobactam	Piperacillin
Escherichia coli	64/65	32/88	16/92	>256/65
Citrobacter koseri	4/94	8/94	4/98	32/90
Citrobacter freundii	>64/60	>64/69	32/84	>64/75
Klebsiella pneumoniae	64/75	16/91	16/91	>256/39
Enterobacter aerogenes	64/44	128/67	128/71	>256/65
Enterobacter cloacae	>256/21	>256/60	>256/69	>256/63
Proteus mirabilis	8/90	2/95	2/96	32/88
Proteus vulgaris	32/46	4/92	4/95	>256/49
Morganella morganii	64/18	32/87	16/91	>256/73
Providencia stuartii	16/57	1/100	2/100	4/100
Serratia marcescens	128/9	32/84	32/87	>256/77
Pseudomonas aeruginosa	>256/2	128/86	64/92	128/89
Acinetobacter baumannii	32/81	>256/74	>256/67	>256/54

Vaccines and Antibiotics

Vaccines and Antibiotics

Table 6.8 Susceptibility of common gram-negative bacilli to selected cephalosporins

Organism	MIC$_{90}$/% susceptible				
	Cefotaxime	Ceftriaxone	Ceftazidime	Cefepime
Escherichia coli	0.25/100	0.25/100	0.25/100	≤0.12/100
Citrobacter koseri	1/100	4/95	0.5/92	0.12/100
Citrobacter freundii	64/64	64/68	>128/71	1/98
Klebsiella pneumoniae	2/95	2/95	2/94	0.25/99
Enterobacter aerogenes	32/75	32/75	16/70	0.25/100
Enterobacter cloacae	128/68	>128/68	128/72	2/100
Proteus mirabilis	≤0.12/100	≤0.12/100	≤0.12/93	≤0.12/100
Proteus vulgaris	64/80	128/88	8/91	0.25/100
Morganella morganii	8/90	1/92	16/80	≤0.12/100
Providencia stuartii	0.5/98	0.5/98	0.25/95	≤0.12/100
Serratia marcescens	16/84	16/87	2/91	1/100
Pseudomonas aeruginosa	>128/12	>128/12	32/88	16/81
Acinetobacter baumannii	>128/38	128/40	32/62	64/69

Table 6.9 Susceptibility of common gram-negative bacilli to imipenem and selected quinolones

Organism	MIC$_{90}$/% susceptible			
	Imipenem	Ciprofloxacin	Levofloxacin	Trovafloxacin
Escherichia coli	≤0.12/100	≤0.12/98	≤0.12/99	≤0.12/99
Citrobacter koseri	≤0.12/100	≤0.12/99	≤0.12/99	≤0.12/99
Citrobacter freundii	0.5/100	≤0.12/91	≤0.12/90	≤0.12/90
Klebsiella pneumoniae	0.5/100	0.5/95	1/94	0.5/95
Enterobacter aerogenes	2/97	0.5/92	0.5/90	0.5/90
Enterobacter cloacae	2/99	0.5/94	0.5/95	0.5/95
Proteus mirabilis	4/97	0.25/97	0.25/99	0.5/98
Proteus vulgaris	4/93	≤0.12/97	≤0.12/98	≤0.12/98
Morganella morganii	8/87	0.25/96	≤0.12/98	0.5/96
Providencia stuartii	2/98	>8/64	>8/62	>8/62
Serratia marcescens	2/99	2/86	2/87	2/87
Pseudomonas aeruginosa	8/88	4/79	8/75	8/75
Acinetobacter baumannii	1/97	16/63	8/65	8/65

Vaccines and Antibiotics

Vaccines and Antibiotics

Table 6.10 Susceptibility patterns for miscellaneous aerobic gram-negative bacteria

Organism	Generally active	Unpredictable activity	Generally inactive
Actinobacillus actinomycetemcomitans	**Cephalosporins**, rifampin, aminoglycosides, tetracycline, chloramphenicol	Penicillins	Erythromycin, clindamycin
Aeromonas hydrophila	**Cephalosporins [broad-spectrum]**, imipenem, quinolones, chloramphenicol	Erythromycin, aminoglycosides, (TMP-SMX[a]), tetracyclines	
Burkholderia cepacia	TMP-SMX	Quinolones	Penicillins, cephalosporins, imipenem
Burkholderia pseudomallei	**Imipenem**, penicillins	Quinolones, cephalosporins [broad-spectrum]	Tetracyclines, chloramphenicol, TMP-SMX
Cardiobacterium hominis	**Penicillin**, cephalosporins, imipenem, chloramphenicol, tetracycline		Aminoglycosides, macrolides, clindamycin
Eikenella corrodens	**Penicillin**, cephalosporins [broad-spectrum], tetracyclines, quinolones	Aminoglycosides	Clindamycin, metronidazole
Haemophilus ducreyi	**Cephalosporins [broad-spectrum]**, quinolones, macrolides	Penicillin, β-lactam–β-lactamase inhibitors, tetracycline, TMP-SMX	
Haemophilus influenzae	**Cephalosporins [broad-spectrum]**, TMP-SMX	Ampicillin, chloramphenicol	
Kingella kingae	**Cephalosporins**, penicillins, imipenem, aminoglycosides, TMP-SMX, erythromycin	Clindamycin	Quinolones

Organism		
Moraxella catarrhalis	**Quinolones**, imipenem, cephalosporins, tetracyclines aminoglycosides, TMP-SMX, macrolides, chloramphenicol	Penicillins
Neisseria gonorrhoeae	**Cephalosporins [broad-spectrum]**	Penicillin, tetracycline, macrolides, quinolones
Pasteurella multocida	**Penicillin**, cephalosporins, imipenem, TMP-SMX, tetracycline, quinolones	Macrolides, clindamycin
Pleisomonas shigelloides	**Cephalosporins**, imipenem, β-lactam–β-lactamase inhibitors, quinolones, aminoglycosides	Penicillins
Stenotrophomonas maltophilia	**TMP-SMX**	Quinolones
Streptobacillus moniliformis	**Penicillin**, tetracycline, chloramphenicol	Penicillins, cephalosporins, imipenem
Vibrio cholerae	**Doxycycline**, TMP-SMX, chloramphenicol	
Vibrio vulnificus	**Doxycycline + cephalosporin [broad-spectrum]**, quinolones	Aminoglycosides

[a]TMP-SMX, trimethoprim-sulfamethoxazole.

Vaccines and Antibiotics

Vaccines and Antibiotics

Table 6.11 Susceptibility patterns for fastidious bacteria

Organism	Generally active	Unpredictable activity	Generally inactive
Bartonella spp.	**Erythromycin, doxycycline**	Penicillins, cephalosporins, imipenem, aminoglycosides, quinolones, TMP-SMX[a]	
Bordetella pertussis	**Erythromycin,** TMP-SMX, quinolones, chloramphenicol		Penicillins, cephalosporins, aminoglycosides
Borrelia burgdorferi	**Doxycycline or cephalosporins [broad-spectrum]**, penicillins, macrolides	Quinolones	Aminoglycosides
Brucella spp.	Doxycycline, TMP-SMX, or quinolones with gentamicin	Cephalosporins	Penicillins
Calymmatobacterium granulomatis	**Tetracyclines,** macrolides, TMP-SMX, chloramphenicol, aminoglycosides, quinolones		Penicillin
Campylobacter spp.	**Macrolides,** tetracycline, chloramphenicol	Quinolones, aminoglycosides	Penicillins, cephalosporins
Coxiella burnetii	**Doxycycline,** quinolones	Chloramphenicol	Penicillins, cephalosporins, imipenem, macrolides, aminoglycosides, TMP-SMX
Chlamydia spp.	**Doxycycline,** erythromycin	Quinolones	Penicillins, cephalosporins, TMP-SMX

Organism			
Ehrlichia spp.	**Doxycycline**, rifampin	Chloramphenicol	Penicillins, cephalosporins, imipenem, macrolides, aminoglycosides
Francisella tularensis	**Streptomycin or gentamicin**, imipenem, quinolones		Penicillins, cephalosporins
Legionella pneumophila	**Erythromycin** or other macrolides, quinolones, rifampin	Tetracycline	
Leptospira interrogans	**Penicillin or doxycycline**, cephalosporins	Penicillins, cephalosporins, aminoglycosides	Chloramphenicol
Mycoplasma pneumoniae	**Macrolides**, tetracyclines	Aminoglycosides, chloramphenicol, quinolones	Penicillins, cephalosporins, imipenem, TMP-SMX
Rickettsia rickettsii	**Doxycycline**, quinolones chloramphenicol	Erythromycin	Penicillins, cephalosporins, imipenem, aminoglycosides, TMP-SMX
Treponema pallidum	**Penicillin**, cephalosporins [broad-spectrum], tetracyclines	Macrolides	Quinolones, rifampin
Ureaplasma urealyticum	**Macrolides**	Clindamycin, tetracyclines, aminoglycosides, quinolones, chloramphenicol	Penicillins, cephalosporins, imipenem, TMP-SMX

[a]TMP-SMX, trimethoprim-sulfamethoxazole.

Vaccines and Antibiotics

Table 6.12 Susceptibility patterns for anaerobic bacteria

Organism	Generally active	Unpredictable activity	Generally inactive
Peptostreptococcus spp.	**Penicillin**, cephalosporins, imipenem, chloramphenicol	Metronidazole, clindamycin	
Actinomyces spp.	**Penicillin**, imipenem	Cephalosporins, clindamycin	
Lactobacillus spp.		Penicillins, cephalosporins, quinolones, vancomycin, metronidazole, clindamycin	Metronidazole
Clostridium perfringens	**Penicillin**, cephalosporins, imipenem, clindamycin, chloramphenicol, metronidazole		
Other *Clostridium* spp.	**Metronidazole or vancomycin**, imipenem, chloramphenicol	Penicillin, cephalosporins, clindamycin	
Bacteroides fragilis	**Metronidazole**, imipenem, β-lactam–β-lactamase inhibitor, chloramphenicol	Clindamycin, cephalosporins [broad-spectrum], cephamycins	Penicillin
Bilophila wadsworthia	**Metronidazole**, chloramphenicol	Clindamycin, imipenem, cephamycins, cephalosporins [broad-spectrum]	Penicillin
Fusobacterium spp.	**Metronidazole**, imipenem, penicillin, clindamycin	Cephalosporins [broad-spectrum], cephamycins	
Mobiluncus spp.	Clindamycin, vancomycin, chloramphenicol, penicillins, cephalosporins, imipenem	Metronidazole	Erythromycin
Porphyromonas spp.	**Metronidazole**, imipenem, chloramphenicol	Cephalosporins [broad-spectrum], cephamycins	Penicillin
Prevotella spp.	**Metronidazole**, imipenem, chloramphenicol	Cephalosporins [broad-spectrum], cephamycins	Penicillin
Veillonella spp.	**Clindamycin**, imipenem, metronidazole	Chloramphenicol	Penicillin, cephalosporins

Table 6.13 Susceptibility patterns for mycobacteria

Organisms	Primary drugs	Secondary drugs
Slowly growing mycobacteria		
M. tuberculosis complex	Isoniazid + rifampin + pyrazinamide + (ethambutol or streptomycin)	*p*-Aminosalicylic acid, ethionamide, cycloserine, capreomycin, kanamycin, amikacin, ciprofloxacin, ofloxacin, rifabutin
M. avium complex	Ethambutol + (clarithromycin or azithromycin) + (clofazimine or rifampin or rifabutin or ciprofloxacin or amikacin)	
M. genavense	As with *M. avium* complex	
M. haemophilum	Clarithromycin + (rifampin or rifabutin) ± other active drugs	Amikacin, ciprofloxacin, doxycycline, TMP-SMX[a]
M. kansasii	Isoniazid + rifampin + ethambutol	Amikacin, streptomycin, ciprofloxacin, clarithromycin, TMP-SMX
M. leprae	Dapsone + rifampin ± clofazimine	Minocycline, clarithromycin, ofloxacin

(continued)

Table 6.13 Susceptibility patterns for mycobacteria *(continued)*

Organisms	Primary drugs	Secondary drugs
M. marinum	Rifampin + ethambutol	Tetracyclines, TMP-SMX
M. malmoense	Isoniazid + rifampin + ethambutol	Cycloserine
M. scrofulaceum	As with *M. avium* complex	
M. szulgai	Isoniazid + rifampin + ethambutol + streptomycin	Amikacin, ciprofloxacin, clarithromycin, TMP-SMX
M. ulcerans	Isoniazid + streptomycin, rifampin + TMP-SMX + minocycline	
M. xenopi	Isoniazid + rifampin + ethambutol, rifampin + streptomycin	
Rapidly growing mycobacteria		
M. abscessus	Amikacin + cefoxitin	Ciprofloxacin, ofloxacin, clarithromycin, azithromycin, TMP-SMX
M. chelonae	Imipenem + amikacin or tobramycin	Clarithromycin, azithromycin
M. fortuitum	Amikacin + cefoxitin	Ciprofloxacin, ofloxacin, clarithromycin, azithromycin, TMP-SMX, imipenem

[a]TMP-SMX, trimethoprim-sulfamethoxazole.

Table 6.14 Susceptibility patterns for viruses

Virus	Antiviral agents
Cytomegalovirus	Foscarnet, ganciclovir, vidarabine, cidofovir
Hepatitis B virus	Foscarnet, interferon
Hepatitis C virus	Interferon
Herpes simplex virus	Acyclovir, foscarnet, ganciclovir, idoxuridine, vidarabine
Human immunodeficiency virus	Protease inhibitor (indinavir or ritonavir or nalfinavir) + zidovudine + lamivudine or didanosine or zalcitabine, protease inhibitor + stavudine + lamivudine or didanosine, zidovudine or stavudine + lamivudine or didanosine or zalcitabine + nevirapine or delavirdine
Influenza A virus	Amantadine, ribavirin, rimantadine
Influenza B virus	Ribavirin
Lassa fever virus	Ribavirin
Papillomavirus	Interferon
Parainfluenza virus	Ribavirin
Respiratory syncytial virus	Ribavirin
Vaccinia virus	Vidarabine
Varicella-zoster virus	Acyclovir, foscarnet, vidarabine

Vaccines and Antibiotics

Vaccines and Antibiotics

Table 6.15 Susceptibility patterns for fungi

Organism	Generally active	Unpredictable activity	Generally inactive
Yeasts			
Candida spp.	Amphotericin B, nystatin, ketoconazole	5-Flucytosine, miconazole, itraconazole, fluconazole	
Cryptococcus neoformans	Amphotericin B + 5-flucytosine, itraconazole	Ketoconazole, miconazole, fluconazole	
Malassezia furfur	Selenium sulfide, miconazole, ketoconazole, itraconazole, amphotericin B		
Trichosporon spp.	Amphotericin B, nystatin, ketoconazole		
Dimorphic fungi			
Blastomyces dermatitidis	Amphotericin B, itraconazole, ketoconazole, miconazole		5-Flucytosine
Coccidioides immitis	Amphotericin B, itraconazole, ketoconazole, miconazole		5-Flucytosine
Histoplasma capsulatum	Amphotericin B, itraconazole, ketoconazole, miconazole		5-Flucytosine

Paracoccidioides brasiliensis	Amphotericin B, itraconazole, fluconazole, sulfonamides	Ketoconazole, miconazole	5-Flucytosine
Sporothrix schenckii	Potassium iodide, intraconazole	Amphotericin B, 5-flucytosine	Ketoconazole, fluconazole
Other molds			
Aspergillus spp.	Amphotericin B, itraconazole	Miconazole, ketoconazole	Fluconazole, 5-flucytosine
Chromoblastomycosis agents[a]	Itraconazole, 5-flucytosine	Miconazole, ketoconazole	Amphotericin B, griseofulvin
Dermatophytes[b]	Miconazole, itraconazole, ketoconazole, clotrimazole, fluconazole, terbinafine, griseofulvin, nystatin		Amphotericin B, 5-flucytosine
Eumycetoma agents[c]	Itraconazole, miconazole	Ketoconazole	Amphotericin B, 5-flucytosine
Zygomycetes[d]	Amphotericin B		Ketoconazole, miconazole, itraconazole, fluconazole, 5-flucytosine

[a]Chromoblastomycosis agents include *Phialophora* and *Cladosporidium* spp.
[b]Dermatophytes include *Epidermophyton, Microsporum,* and *Trichophyton* spp.
[c]Eumycetoma agents include *Madurella, Pseudallescheria,* and *Cephalosporium* spp.
[d]Zygomycetes include *Mucor, Rhizopus,* and *Absidia* spp.

Vaccines and Antibiotics

Table 6.16 Susceptibility patterns for parasites

Parasites	Antiparasitic agents
Protozoa	
Babesia microti	Clindamycin + quinine
Balantidium coli	Metronidazole, tetracycline, iodoquinol
Cryptosporidium parvum	Paromomycin
Cyclospora cayetanensis	TMP-SMX[a]
Dientamoeba fragilis	Iodoquinol, tetracycline
Entamoeba histolytica	Metronidazole
Giardia lamblia	Metronidazole, albendazole, quinacrine
Isospora belli	TMP-SMX
Leishmania spp.	Sodium stibogluconate (CDC), meglumine antimonate, amphotericin B, pentamidine
Microsporidia	Albendazole
Naegleria fowleri	Amphotericin B
Plasmodium falciparum	
Chloroquine resistant	Quinine + fansidar or tetracycline
Chloroquine susceptible	Cloroquine, quinidine
Other *Plasmodium* spp.	Chloroquine or quinidine + primaquine
Toxoplasma gondii	Fansidar, spiramycin
Trichomonas vaginalis	Metronidazole
Trypanosoma cruzi	Nifurtimox, benznidazole
Trypanosoma brucei	Suramin (CDC), melarsoprol (CDC), pentamidine
Cestodes	
Cysticercus cellulosae	Albendazole, praziquantel
Echinococcus spp.	Albendazole
Intestinal tapeworms	Praziquantel, niclosamide
Nematodes	
Dracunculus medinensis	Metronidazole, thiabendazole
Enterobius vermicularis	Pyrantel, mebendazole, albendazole, ivermectin
Filaria	
Onchocerca volvulus	Ivermectin (CDC)
All others	Diethylcarbamazine
Hookworm	Mebendazole, pyrantel, albendazole

(continued)

Table 6.16 Susceptibility patterns for parasites (*continued*)

Parasites	Antiparasitic agents
Strongyloides stercoralis	Thiabendazole, albendazole, ivermectin
Toxocara spp.	Diethylcarbamazine, albendazole, mebendazole
Trichostrongylus spp.	Pyrantel, mebendazole, albendazole
Trichuris trichiura	Mebendazole, albendazole, ivermectin
Others	Mebendazole, pyrantel, albendazole, ivermectin
Trematodes	
Fasciola hepatica	Bithionol (CDC), triclabendazole
Schistosoma spp.	Praziquantel, oxamniquine
All others	Praziquantel

[a]TMP-SMX, trimethoprim-sulfamethoxazole.

Immunodiagnostic Tests

Diagnostic tests are divided into two general categories: tests to detect an organism, its antigens, metabolic by-products, or genetic material; and tests to measure the patient's immune response to the infection. Antigen detection tests can be used with a variety of specimens including blood or serum, cerebrospinal fluid, other normally sterile fluids, urine, and tissue. Antibody detection tests are performed primarily with serum or plasma specimens. Whereas the presence of an antigen in a clinical specimen can be interpreted with relative ease, monitoring a patient's humoral immune response is more complex. The presence of antibodies directed against an organism can represent active disease, asymptomatic colonization, or an infection in the recent or distant past. Although high levels or titers of antibodies can be indicative of current infection, most diagnostic procedures require demonstration of a significant increase or decrease in antibodies (e.g., a fourfold or greater change in antibody titer). Interpretation of antibody detection tests is also complicated by the testing method and the patient population under evaluation. For these reasons, general interpretive guidelines are useful but must be supplemented with knowledge of the limitations of the specific test method and other testing variables that influence the requested test.

This chapter contains a review of the diagnostic tests for the most common bacterial, viral, fungal, and parasitic infections. Tests used to detect the organisms, as well as the patient's immune response to the infections, are listed. It should be recognized that the status of diagnostic testing continues to evolve. For example, molecular diagnostic tests are currently available for many microbes but, with only a few exceptions, most of these tests are not widely available. However, the technology is rapidly evolving, and it is expected that many tests that are currently stated to be available only in research laboratories will be used routinely in the near future.

A number of abbreviations of test procedures are used throughout this section. The following is a definition of these terms. ACIF, anticomplementary immunofluorescence; CF, complement fixation; CIE, counterimmunoelectrophoresis; DFA, direct fluorescent antibody; EIA, enzyme immunoassay; ELISA, enzyme-linked immunosorbent assay; FA, fluorescent-antibody test; FIA, fluorescence immunoassay;

HAI, hemagglutination inhibition; ID, immunodiffusion; IFA, indirect fluorescent-antibody test; IHA, indirect hemagglutination; LA, latex agglutination; LCR, ligase chain reaction; MAT, microscopic agglutination test; micro-IF, microimmunofluorescence test; NT, neutralization test; RIA, radioimmunoassay; RIPA, radioimmunoprecipitation assay; RT-PCR, reverse transcriptase-PCR; TA, tube agglutination; TMA, transcription-mediated amplification; TP, tube precipitin.

Immunodiagnostic Tests: Interpretive Values

Bacteria

***Actinomyces* spp.** The clinical diagnosis of actinomycosis is confirmed by microscopic examination of clinical specimens and isolation of the anaerobic organism in culture. Direct FA can augment Gram stain for initial detection. Serological testing is not helpful.

***Bartonella henselae* (Bartonellosis; Cat Scratch Disease).** *Bartonella henselae* can be cultured in patients with bacteremia, bacillary angiomatosis, and bacillary peliosis but rarely in patients with cat scratch disease. PCR has also been used and may become the diagnostic method of choice, but currently it is restricted to research investigations. At present, the most useful method is serological testing. Although hemagglutination and IFA assays have been developed, EIA is the test of choice. The test has high sensitivity (95%) and specificity (>95%) for cat scratch disease, with immunoglobulin M (IgM) antibodies developing early in disease and IgG antibodies developing later. Immunocompetent patients with endocarditis also have highly elevated antibody titers. Cross-reactions with *Coxiella* and *Chlamydia* spp. occur but generally at only a low level. The value of serological testing in immunocompromised patients (e.g., HIV-infected patients) is less clear; however, large numbers of organisms are typically present, facilitating isolation in culture or detection by microscopy.

***Bordetella pertussis* (Pertussis).** Infections with *Bordetella pertussis* are typically confirmed by microscopy (i.e., FA) or culture. The sensitivity and specificity of FA (and serological testing) are unknown because culture is fraught with problems. Assays for *B. pertussis* antigens (e.g., pertussis toxin [PT] and filamentous hemagglutinin [FHA]) have been developed but are not commonly used. PCR assays have been developed and may become the definitive diagnostic tests. However, at present, the diagnosis of pertussis is frequently validated by serological testing. Although many different test methods have been evaluated, ELISA appears to be the most promising and popular. The test has a high sensitivity for detection of increases in antibody titers in paired sera when antibodies to several antigens are measured (e.g., IgG to FHA and PT; IgA to FHA). *Haemophilus influenzae* antigens are serologically related to FHA, and so cross-reactions can occur. Tests for IgA antibodies show promise as rapid diagnostic tests because IgA antibodies are not produced after immunization and are detected only during the acute phase of illness. Antibody titers develop slowly and are not detected until 1 to 2 weeks after the onset of disease. IgA and IgM titers decline to low levels within 3 to 5 months, while the IgG titer remains elevated for much longer.

***Borrelia* Species (Relapsing Fever).**   Relapsing fever is diagnosed primarily by direct observation of spirochetes in peripheral blood smears prepared during a febrile episode (70% sensitivity). Alternatively, diagnosis is confirmed by culture or serological testing. Many species of relapsing fever spirochetes are not available for preparation of antigens in serological tests. Additionally, spontaneous changes of surface antigens in the spirochetes also make serodiagnosis difficult. However, promising results have been obtained with cultured spirochetes as antigens in IFA, ELISA, and immunoblot assays. A titer of 1:64 or greater by IFA is considered positive, although cross-reactions with other spirochetes occur.

***Borrelia burgdorferi* (Lyme Disease).**   Lyme disease is a clinical diagnosis that can be proven by microscopic detection or recovery of *Borrelia burgdorferi* (or other implicated species). Serological tests can confirm the clinical diagnosis but are not diagnostic by themselves. IgM and IgG antibodies can be detected by ELISA or IFA, and these results can be confirmed by immunoblot analysis. Interpretation of serological tests for Lyme disease is complicated by the observation that significant cross-reactivity has been observed in patients infected with other species of

Borrelia; in patients with syphilis, leptospirosis, or periodontal disease; and in patients with infectious mononucleosis, bacterial endocarditis, or autoimmune disease. At the time of initial disease manifestations (i.e., erythema migrans), positive IgM or IgG antibodies will be detected in fewer than 50% of patients. Antibiotic therapy early in the course of disease may also reduce antibody responses. However, patients with late manifestations (e.g., arthritis, neuroborreliosis, or carditis) typically have high antibody titers. Significant variations in commercial reagents and technological performance of the test contribute to sensitivity and specificity problems. Efforts to purify species-specific antigens have identified a 39-kDa protein which is conserved among all Lyme disease spirochetes and may resolve specificity problems with this assay. A positive IgM immunoassay is confirmed by immunoblotting by detecting at least two of three bacterial proteins (21 to 25, 39, and 41 kDa). IgG immunoassays are confirmed by detecting at least 5 of 10 proteins (18, 21 to 25, 28, 30, 39, 41, 45, 58, 66, and 93 kDa).

***Brucella* Species (Brucellosis).** *Brucella* spp. are rarely observed by microscopy; therefore, clinical diagnosis is confirmed by either culture or serological testing. Tube agglutination or microagglutination tests are most commonly performed. A titer of 1:160 or greater is consistent with disease. However, elevated levels of antibodies in serum are common in individuals living in areas of endemic infection; cross-reactions occur with many organisms (e.g., *Salmonella*, *Francisella*, and *Vibrio* spp.), lupus, and myeloma; and many patients will fail to mount an immune response. Thus, the diagnosis of brucellosis should not rest on serological testing alone.

***Chlamydia* Species.** *Chlamydia* infections have historically been confirmed by culture, observation of elementary bodies in specimens by DFA, or detection of chlamydial antigens (i.e., lipopolysaccharide [LPS] and major outer membrane protein [MOMP]) by EIA. More recently, these methods have been replaced by molecular methods, initially probe tests and now amplification tests, including PCR, LCR, and TMA. Amplification tests are the most sensitive method; however, they are currently approved only for genital specimens. Two serological tests are in gen-

Immunodiagnostic Tests

eral use: CF and micro-IF. The CF test is genus specific, detecting antibodies to all three pathogenic species: *C. trachomatis*, *C. psittaci*, and *C. pneumoniae*. The micro-IF test is type specific, requiring the use of multiple antigens to broaden its reactivity. The CF test is positive in virtually all patients with psittacosis or lymphogranuloma venereum (LGV); occasionally positive in patients with *C. pneumoniae* infection, inclusion conjunctivitis, or cervical infection; and generally not positive in patients with oculogenital infections and trachoma. A positive CF titer is 1:16 or greater. CF titers for patients with LGV or psittacosis generally exceed 1:128, while patients with inclusion conjunctivitis, cervicitis, or urethritis have antibody titers of <1:16. Titers in asymptomatic patients vary widely depending upon the disease prevalence in the population. The micro-IF test is more sensitive than the CF test. Most patients with chlamydial infections have positive reactivity (90 to 100% of patients have detectable IgG antibodies; IgM antibodies are less common). However, antibodies to past infections persist for years and are commonly detected in the assay. Infants with *C. trachomatis* pneumonia invariably have high IgM antibody levels (1:128 or greater).

***Clostridium botulinum* Toxin.**   The Centers for Disease Control and Prevention (CDC) provides tests measuring the level of antibodies against *C. botulinum* toxin (antitoxin levels) in patients immunized with toxoid. These tests assess immunity and cannot be used for the diagnosis of botulism. The appropriate diagnostic test for food-borne botulism is demonstration of botulinal toxin in serum, feces, gastric contents, or vomitus or recovery of the organism in the feces of the patient. Demonstration of the organism or toxin in suspected foods provides indirect evidence of botulism. The presence of the organism or detection of toxin in wound exudates confirms the diagnosis of wound botulism.

***Clostridium tetani* Toxin.**   The mouse protection assay is the definitive test to demonstrate antibodies against *C. tetani* toxin (antitoxin levels) in patients immunized with toxoid. Alternative laboratory-based tests include ELISA, CIE, and RIA. ELISA is the most sensitive and reproducible of these tests but should be used only for screening and not for determination of the specific antibody titer. ELISA assesses immunity and cannot be used for the diagnosis of tetanus. Toxin levels of ≥0.5 IU/ml are generally considered protective. Lower levels indicate that immunization with toxoid may be required. The diagnosis of tetanus is based on clinical parameters; laboratory testing has minimal value.

***Corynebacterium diphtheriae* Toxin.**   EIAs have been developed to measure the level of antibodies against *C. diphtheriae* toxin (antitoxin levels) in patients immunized with toxoid. This test assesses immunity and cannot be used for the diagnosis of diphtheria. Toxin levels of ≥0.01 IU/ml are considered protective. Lower levels indicate that immunization with toxoid may be required. The diagnosis of diphtheria is based on clinical parameters and the recovery of toxin-producing strains of *C. diphtheriae* from clinical specimens.

***Coxiella burnetii* (Q Fever).**   *C. burnetii* can be recovered in culture, although this is rarely attempted. PCR appears to be sensitive but is currently restricted to research laboratories. A variety of serological methods, including microagglutination, CF, IFA, and ELISA, have been used. Indirect IFA is currently the method of choice. ELISA appears to be more sensitive than IFA, but interpretive standards have not been defined. Antigenic phase variation occurs with *C. burnetii* infections. In acute self-limited infections, antibodies to the phase II antigen appear first and dominate the immune response. In chronic infections, antibody titers to phase I antigen predominate. Phase II antibodies appear first and peak within 1 month at 1:1,024 or 1:2,048. Phase I antibodies appear later and peak at 4 months. The ratio between phase I and phase II responses may be useful for distinguishing between acute and chronic infections. A phase I titer of 1:800 or greater is diagnostic for chronic Q fever (e.g., endocarditis).

***Ehrlichia* Species.**   The two most common forms of human ehrlichiosis are human monocytic ehrlichiosis (HME), caused by *E. chaffeensis*, and human granulocytic ehrlichiosis (HGE), an infection recently attributed to an unnamed ehrlichia in the *E. phagocytophila* group. Although both organisms have been cultured, this is rarely done in the clinical laboratory. Infected peripheral blood cells can also be detected with Giemsa stain or immunohistological stains, but these procedures are relatively insensitive. PCR assays have been developed; although they are currently restricted to research laboratories, these methods are likely to become the test of choice. Most infections are currently diagnosed serologically by IFA. A fourfold change in titer or a convalescent-phase titer of 1:64 or greater is consistent with the diagnosis of HME. Cross-reactivity has been reported in patients with Rocky Mountain spotted fever, Q fever, brucellosis, Lyme disease, and Epstein-Barr virus infections. These can be resolved by confirming IFA results with immunoblots (detection of *E. chaffeensis*-specific 22-, 28-, 29-, or 120-kDa antigens). HME is confirmed by detecting antibodies by the IFA test at a 1:64 or greater dilution of the patient's serum. The specificity of the assay is demonstrated by detecting antibodies to the 44-kDa *E. phagocytophila* group antigen.

Escherichia coli.   Although culture is the most common method for detecting *E. coli* infections, a variety of antigen tests have been developed. The heat-labile and heat-stable toxins of enterotoxigenic *E. coli* can be detected by ELISA and DNA probe tests. Likewise, ELISA and agglutination assays are available for detecting the Shiga-like toxin of enterohemorrhagic *E. coli* (EHEC). Antibodies against the toxin and LPS antigen of EHEC can also be detected by ELISA, with antibody titers peaking 2 to 3 weeks after the initial infection (at the time when hemolytic-uremic syndrome develops).

***Francisella tularensis* (Tularemia).**   The diagnosis of tularemia can be confirmed by microscopy (i.e., IFA) or culture. However, in laboratories inexperienced with *F. tularensis*, serological testing can be used to support the clinical diagnosis. Although the microagglutination test is the most sensitive assay, the tube agglutination test is most commonly used. Antibody titers are generally negative in the first week of illness, become positive by the end of the second week, and peak after 4 to 5 weeks. A fourfold or greater increase in antibody titer or a single agglutination titer of ≥1:160 is considered diagnostic of active or recent infection. Elevated antibody titers late in disease are common, and levels from 1:20 to 1:80 may persist for years. Antibody titers of <1:20 usually represent nonspecific cross-reactions. Cross-reactivity with *Legionella* antigens can occur.

Immunodiagnostic Tests

***Haemophilus* Species.** *H. influenzae* can be easily recovered in culture, so other tests are less important. Previously, detection of type-specific capsular antigens was used to facilitate the diagnosis of disseminated disease (e.g., meningitis); however, this test is no more sensitive than a Gram stain, and vaccination has dramatically reduced the incidence of *H. influenzae* disease. PCR-based tests have also been developed but are rarely used. Serological testing is now generally restricted to demonstration of a response to vaccination. DFA and EIA have been developed for detecting *H. ducreyi* antigens, as well as PCR-based DNA assays. Further evaluation of these tests is required before they can be accepted for use. Measurement of IgG and IgM antibodies by EIA has also been described for *H. ducreyi*, but the test sensitivity and specificity are poor.

Helicobacter pylori. The urease test (e.g., CLO test, the urea breath test) is the most rapid, sensitive method for detecting *H. pylori*. PCR assays have also been developed but offer few advantages over the urease tests. Elevated IgM, IgG, and IgA titers are also associated with *H. pylori* infections. These antibodies have been measured by CF, hemagglutination, immunoblotting, FIA, and ELISA, with ELISA found to be the most useful. IgM measurement is not clinically useful. Measurement of IgG and IgA antibody titers can be used to diagnose active disease (screen with IgG assay; resolve equivocal reactions with IgA assay). Elevated antibody levels are present in many adult patients; therefore, diagnosis of active disease is dependent upon detection of a fourfold or greater increase in antibody titer. The test sensitivity is generally >95% and the specificity is >90% (highest when purified antigens are used in the reaction). Antibody levels decrease >20% over a 6-month period in successfully treated patients.

***Legionella pneumophila* (Legionellosis).** Infections are most commonly diagnosed by culture. DFA has been used to detect *L. pneumophila* and *L. micdadei* (25 to 75% sensitivity; 90% specificity). RIA, EIA, and LA assays have been developed to detect *L. pneumophila* serogroup 1 antigens in urine. The urine test is sensitive and specific but cannot detect other serogroups or species. Antigen can be excreted for months after successful treatment. PCR tests are currently available only for environmental samples.

Measurement of antibody response (by immunofluorescence, ELISA, or RIA) requires demonstration of seroconversion. No single titer is now considered diagnostic. A fourfold or greater rise in antibody titer to at least ≥1:128 is indicative of active infection. Some patients (20 to 30%) fail to produce a diagnostic antibody response. Patients who seroconvert will do so within 9 to 10 weeks, with 75% documented to seroconvert in the first 3 weeks. The specificity is greater than 95%, but cross-reactions with a variety of gram-negative and gram-positive bacteria (e.g., *Campylobacter* and *Pseudomonas* spp.) have been observed.

***Leptospira* Species (Leptospirosis).** *Leptospira* species can be cultured from blood and cerebrospinal fluid (CSF) during the first 10 days of illness and in urine after the first week. Dark-field microscopy or DFA tests can be used to detect the organisms in clinical specimens or culture. PCR assays have also been developed. Antibodies are detected after 1 week of illness, with peak titers at 3 to 4 weeks postinfection. The MAT is sensitive and specific and is used as the reference test for less cumbersome methods. A positive test is defined as a fourfold or greater rise in antibodies (may require 1 month or longer). A titer of 1:200 is suggestive, and a titer of 1:800 or greater is considered definitive. Cross-reactions occur with other spirochetes and with *Legionella* species. Other assays (genus specific) include slide agglutination, IHA, CF, and ELISA. Currently the ELISA is the most sensitive and specific. An IHA antibody titer of ≥1:100 is considered indicative of active or recent infection. However, this genus-specific test is considered relatively insensitive. CF can be used to determine subgroup specificity, but it also lacks sensitivity.

Listeria monocytogenes. The diagnosis of listeriosis is confirmed by isolation of the organism in culture. PCR tests have been developed in research laboratories, and preliminary reports indicate that they are highly sensitive and specific. Serological tests are not useful.

Mycobacterium tuberculosis. Tuberculosis is most commonly diagnosed by microscopy (acid-fast stain) or culture. Direct detection of mycobacteria has also been accomplished by using DNA probes (too insensitive except for identification of isolated bacilli) and molecular amplification methods (e.g., PCR, LCR, TMA, and strand displace-

Immunodiagnostic Tests

ment). The amplification methods are useful for smear-positive respiratory specimens but cannot be used for non-respiratory or smear-negative specimens. Antigen capture tests (i.e., ELISA, RIA, and agglutination) with purified antigens (i.e., 38-kDa antigen, lipoarabinomannan, antigen 60, and antigen 85 complex) have been developed but are not widely used and cannot replace traditional methods. Serological methods, with the exception of the skin test for cellular immunity, have not proved to be useful.

Mycoplasma pneumoniae. Culture isolation of *M. pneumoniae* is slow and insensitive. For this reason, a variety of antigen-directed tests, including DFA, EIA, and immunoblotting, have been developed. These tests, as well as DNA probes, have poor sensitivity and specificity. In contrast, PCR amplification is reported to be highly sensitive and specific. Specific serological tests include CF, ELISA, IFA, and LA. CF primarily detects IgM antibodies. Fourfold or greater increases in antibody titer are observed for about 60% of culture-positive patients, while 80 to 90% of patients will have a single titer of >1:32. ELISA detects either IgM or IgG antibodies and appears to be more sensitive than CF. Specificity can be improved by using purified P1 adhesin protein as the capture antigen. Immunofluorescence IgG and IgM antibody titers of ≥1:10 are considered positive, with active disease indicated by the presence of IgM antibodies or a fourfold or greater rise in the IgG antibody titer. The LA assay detects IgG and IgM antibodies. A single agglutination antibody titer of ≥1:320 or a fourfold or greater rise in antibody titer is indicative of active or recent infection. The specificity of each of these test is a problem because cross-reactions with other *Mycoplasma* species have been observed.

Neisseria gonorrhoeae. *N. gonorrhoeae* can be presumptively detected by ELISA (Gonozyme). However, all positive reactions must be confirmed by culture because cross-reactions with saprophytic bacteria (e.g., neisseriae, *Moraxella catarrhalis*, and *Bacteroides*, *Peptostreptococcus*, *Enterobacter*, and *Proteus* spp.) can occur. Culture of genital specimens and use of immunoassays have now been replaced by molecular tests, initially with rRNA probes and more recently with amplification methods (e.g., PCR, LCR, and TMA). These tests can be used with cervical, urethral,

Immunodiagnostic Tests

and urine specimens and are more sensitive than culture or immunoassays. Antibody testing for the diagnosis of gonococcal disease has not proven to be useful.

Neisseria meningitidis. LA, coagglutination, CIE, and EIA have been developed to detect meningococcal antigens in patients with meningitis and other disseminated infections. LA and EIA have a sensitivity approaching 90% for serogroups A, C, Y, and W135 but a much lower sensitivity for serogroup B. Cross-reaction occurs between serogroup B and *E. coli* K1, as well as between serogroup B and *Moraxella nonliquefaciens.* A PCR assay for meningococcal DNA in CSF has been developed but is not commercially available.

***Nocardia* Species.** Diagnosis of nocardiosis relies upon microscopic detection of the organism in clinical specimens and isolation in culture. Serological methods have been handicapped by the antigenic heterogeneity of pathogenic *Nocardia* spp., poor serological response of the patient, high levels of immunoreactivity to *Nocardia* spp. in healthy individuals, and cross-reactivity with other microbial antigens.

Rickettsia rickettsii. Members of the spotted fever group of rickettsiae can be detected in tissue specimens by immunofluorescence or PCR. It is likely that PCR will become the diagnostic test of choice with greater experience and more widespread availability. A variety of group-specific serological tests have been developed (e.g., IFA, CF, ELISA, RIA, LA, and hemagglutination). Immunofluorescence IgG antibody titers of ≥1:64 are considered indicative of exposure to *Rickettsia rickettsii*. A fourfold or greater rise in titer generally occurs after 3 weeks or more and is consistent with active or recent infection.

Rickettsia typhi. Infection with the typhus group of rickettsiae is confirmed by serological testing. Extensive cross-reactions occur among members of this group; therefore, identification of the specific rickettsia is determined by the clinical presentation of disease. The diagnostic test of choice is either IFA or micro-IF. Immunofluorescence IgG antibody titers of ≥1:64 are considered indicative of exposure to *Rickettsia typhi*. A fourfold or greater rise in antibody titer is indicative of active or recent infection.

Immunodiagnostic Tests

***Salmonella* spp.** The Widal agglutination test measures antibodies to the H and O antigens of *S. typhi* and *S. paratyphi*. IgM is primarily measured; titers peak at 2 to 3 weeks after exposure and do not persist. At a serum dilution of 1:160, the test has a sensitivity of 46% and a specificity of 98%. The test sensitivity improves at lower dilutions, but the specificity is unacceptably low. Cross-reactivity with other group D *Salmonella* spp. occurs. IgG and IgM ELISAs (against both O and Vi antigens) have also been developed but are not widely used.

***Streptococcus*, Group A.** Numerous direct antigen tests (ELISA, DFA, and LA) are available for streptococcal pharyngitis. Although the tests are highly specific, negative reactions must be confirmed by culture (sensitivity, <80%). Antibody tests are used to confirm antecedent group A streptococcal pharyngitis or pyoderma in patients with suspected rheumatic fever or nephritis. The most popular tests are anti-streptolysin O (ASO) and anti-DNase B. Both tests have a sensitivity of 85%, and they should be performed together. The ASO test is nonreactive in patients with nephritis following streptococcal pyoderma. False-positive ASO titers can occur in patients with liver disease and infections with streptococcal groups C or G. Anti-DNase B is specific for group A streptococci; there is no reaction with other streptococcal groups. Peak ASO and anti-DNase B titers occur 2 to 3 weeks after the primary infection and persist for 6 months or more. Positive titers are 2 or more dilutions above the upper limit of normal. Other tests (e.g., Streptozyme) are less sensitive and reproducible.

***Streptococcus*, Group B.** Numerous direct antigen tests (ELISA, LA) have been developed for group B streptococcal infections, primarily in pregnant women. Although these tests are rapid, they have a sensitivity of <75% and are currently not recommended unless used with culture.

Streptococcus pneumoniae. LA, coagglutination, and CIE have been used to detect pneumococcal antigens in CSF and urine (these tests are less sensitive with urine than with CSF). The tests are generally no more sensitive than a Gram stain and are not currently used in most laboratories. Type-specific anticapsular antibodies can be measured to assess the response to vaccination but are not assayed for diagnostic purposes.

Treponema pallidum **(Syphilis).** Refer to Table 7.1.

Yersinia **Species.** Antibodies against the F1 capsular antigen of *Y. pestis* can be assayed by ELISA at the CDC. A titer of 1:10 is presumptive evidence of infection; however, some patients have little or no response. Infection with *Y. enterocolitica* or *Y. pseudotuberculosis* can be detected by ELISA, microhemagglutination, CF, or immunoblotting for specific antibodies.

Viruses

Adenovirus. Numerous tests are available to document adenovirus infections; they include culture, direct examination by electron microscopy, immunoassays for viral antigens (IFA, RIA, and CIE), PCR amplification, and serological testing. CF and EIA can measure viral genus-specific antibodies, and HAI and NT tests can measure type-specific antibodies. The CF test is cumbersome and less sensitive than the other tests, and EIAs have not been adequately standardized. Although HAI and NT tests are type specific, a heterotypic response to related adenoviruses can occur. Thus, definitive classification of the virus requires isolation in culture. A fourfold or greater rise in antibody titer is required to demonstrate active or recent infection. IgM antibody titers can be measured by EIA, but the sensitivity of the test is low, and so it cannot replace IgG antibody tests.

California Encephalitis Virus. A positive FA antibody titer is ≥1:8. A fourfold or greater rise in titer is indicative of active or recent infection.

Cytomegalovirus. Infections with cytomegalovirus (CMV) can be demonstrated by culture, microscopy, antigen tests, and molecular hybridization. Culture is slow and insensitive compared with new diagnostic methods but provides definitive proof of infection. Microscopic methods for directly detecting virus-infected cells include the use of histopathological stains (e.g., Giemsa, hematoxylin-eosin, and Papanicolaou) and FA. A new variation of FA involves monoclonal antibodies directed against the 65-kDa viral phosphoprotein (pp65) found in the nuclei of peripheral blood leukocytes. The pp65 antigen test is a very sensitive assay for viral replication, and quantitation of the antigen may have prognostic value. Immunoblotting, in situ hybridization, and PCR amplification have each been used. PCR is highly sensitive and may become the diagnostic test of choice for documenting CMV infection. A variety of serological tests have been used to document CMV infection. CF is relatively insensitive and has been replaced in most laboratories by EIA. Other methods include IFA, ACIF, IHA, and neutralization. IHA is reliable for differentiating IgM and IgG antibodies, and neutralization is used to demonstrate strain differences among isolates. However, neither of these assays is commercially available; they are used primarily in research laboratories. A variety of commercially prepared EIAs are available and can be used to quantitate IgM and IgG antibodies, as well as IgG subclasses. IFA and ACIF are used to measure IgM and IgG antibodies, respectively. False-positive IgM reactions occur with patients with Epstein-Barr virus or varicella infections or rheumatoid factor (RF). Cross-reactivity between CMV and human herpesvirus 6 can also occur. The presence of RF should be determined by a sensitive assay (not slide agglutination) or removed (not with protein A). False-negative IgM assays in newborns can also be caused by high maternal IgG titers. IgM antibodies are detected during primary infection, as well as during reactivated disease. Therefore, detection of IgM does not distinguish between these states.

Dengue Virus.   Both IgM and IgG antibodies against all four dengue fever virus types can be detected by the FA assay. Cross-reacting IgG antibodies are observed among all four types. In most patients, dengue antibodies are detectable a week after the onset of symptoms. Cross-reactivity with other arboviruses can occur.

Eastern Equine Encephalitis Virus.   Antibody titers of ≥1:8 are considered positive in the FA assay. A fourfold or greater rise in antibody titer indicates active or recent infection.

Enteroviruses. The most direct way to demonstrate infection with the enteroviruses (i.e., poliovirus, cocksackieviruses, and echovirus) is culture. However, some viruses are difficult to cultivate, and alternative testing methods are required. Unfortunately, in the absence of shared antigens, immunoassays have not proven to be useful. RT-PCR has been used but at present is limited primarily to research laboratories. Serological testing also has limitations. NT, CF, and HAI tests have been developed. Neutralizing antibodies develop early in infection and persist for life, and so it is difficult to demonstrate a significant increase in antibody titer. CF tests are also of limited value because the antibodies are short-lived and cross-react with many members of the enterovirus group. Many enteroviruses fail to hemagglutinate erythrocytes, and so the HAI test has limited value.

Epstein-Barr Virus (Infectious Mononucleosis). A variety of tests have been developed to detect Epstein-Barr virus (EBV) or viral antigens in tissue and peripheral blood. Although techniques for viral culture exist, they are rarely used because patients with latent infections may shed virus during asymptomatic phases and culture is technically cumbersome. IFA and EIA have been used to detect viral latent antigens (EBNA-2 and membrane protein LMP), early antigens (EA p50, Ea p85, EA p17, and BZLF1), and late antigens (VCA p160 and VCA gp125) in clinical specimens. Nucleic acid methods (immunoblotting, PCR, and DNA hybridization) have been used to detect EBV DNA in clinical specimens. PCR is the most sensitive method and is likely to become the test of choice for demonstrating viral infection. Serological testing has been the major method for documenting EBV infections. Infections are common, as indicated by positive Paul-Bunnell heterophile antibody tests in more than 85% of the population; 2 to 3% of patients have false-positive reactivity (many of these cases are attributed to technical error). False-negative reactivity is reported for 10% of adult patients and as many as 50% of pediatric patients. For these patients, EBV-specific testing is required to differentiate between EBV infections and similar clinical disease caused by CMV, adenovirus, and *Toxoplasma gondii*. Immunofluorescence and neutralization tests and EIA are used to detect EBV latent, early, and late antigens. The antibody profiles for patients with different stages of EBV infection are summarized in Table 7.2.

Hantavirus. Hantaviruses are the etiologic agents of hemorrhagic fever with renal syndrome. Antibodies produced by patients with this infection usually cross-react with other viruses in the family. Active or recent infection is suggested by an elevated antibody titer (e.g., $\geq$1:1,024) or a fourfold or greater increase in titer.

Immunodiagnostic Tests

Hepatitis A Virus.   The diagnosis of acute or past infection with hepatitis A virus is assessed by measuring IgM and total antibody titers by EIA. IgM antibodies directed against the virus are almost always present in the patient's serum at the time when symptoms develop. A total antibody response (IgM, IgG, and IgA) develops during the acute phase and persists indefinitely. The presence of IgM alone is consistent with active, acute disease. IgM antibody with a positive total-antibody titer is consistent with either active or recent disease; and a positive total-antibody titer but negative IgM antibody is consistent with a past infection and represents immunity.

Hepatitis B Virus.   Infection with hepatitis B virus (HBV) is demonstrated by detection of virus-specific antigens (surface antigen [HBsAg], core antigen, and e antigen) or antibodies to these antigens. EIA and RIA are most commonly used to measure the levels of these antigens and antibodies. Refer to Table 7.3 for interpretation of HBV tests.

Hepatitis C Virus.   HCV diagnosis is currently achieved by detecting specific antibody by EIA and immunoblot assays that use antigens derived from cloning the HCV genome. If both antibody tests are positive, there is a high likelihood that the patient is infected. The virus can also be detected by RT-PCR or alternative genomic amplification tests.

Hepatitis D Virus.   The duration of HBV infection determines the duration of HDV infection. IgM antibodies directed against HDV are transient during acute infection, and IgG antibodies are often undetectable once the HBsAg disappears.

Herpes Simplex Virus. Infection with herpes simplex virus (HSV) can be documented by culture, microscopy, immunoassays, and PCR. Virus-infected cells can be observed with the Papanicolaou stain or Tzanck test, but these are insensitive and are not specific for HSV. DFA has a sensitivity between 78 and 90%. ELISA, immunoperoxidase assay, and HAI assays have sensitivities between 70 and 95% and specificities between 65 and 95%. PCR testing has proven valuable for documenting central nervous system infections and genital infections with HSV. Serological tests measuring the levels of antibodies against HSV include IFA, EIA, NT, IHA inhibition, and immunoblotting. Cross-reactivity occurs between HSV-1 and HSV-2, and so serological testing does not readily distinguish between the two viruses. The presence of IgM antibodies or a fourfold rise in IgG antibody titer indicates active or recent infection; however, increases in antibody titer do not always occur in patients with recurrent disease, particularly in asymptomatic patients shedding the virus. Cross-reactivity occurs with varicella-zoster virus (VZV) but not with other human herpesviruses. Antigens for both HSV and VZV must be used to determine which virus is responsible for the antibody response. IFA tests have been associated with nonspecific reactions. This is minimized by using the anticomplement IFA method. However, this method is rarely used now and has been replaced by EIA. Type-specific EIAs can be performed if the gG1 and gG2 antigens are used. However, these are not widely available at present. Although claims are made that the NT test is type specific, HSV-2 antibodies cannot be reliably identified. The IHA inhibition test is type specific if type-specific antigens are used to remove homologous antibodies selectively.

Human Herpesvirus 6. Diagnostic tests for human herpesvirus 6 (HHV-6) include culture, microscopy, detection of viral DNA, and serological tests. Culture is slow, requiring detection of viral antigens in infected cells by IFA, ACIF, or EIA. IFA has been used to detect viral antigens in clinical specimens. In situ hybridization and PCR have also been used to detect viruses in specimens. Tests used for the serodiagnosis of HHV-6 infections include IFA, ACIF, EIA, and NT. IFA is the most widely used method; although historically it has been plagued with sensitivity and specificity problems, recent improvements in the preparation of test antigens have helped solve these problems. ACIF was originally developed to compensate for the problems with IFA. This test is now used to measure IgG antibody titers. EIAs can detect both IgG and IgM antibodies, although the accuracy of this EIA needs to be demonstrated. NTs are comparable to EIA but are rarely used because of technical difficulties. As with the other herpesvirus infections, IgM antibodies appear in primary infections, persist for months, and can be found in patients with reactivated disease. Fourfold or greater increases in IgG antibody titers can indicate active disease. However, this may be difficult to demonstrate, particularly during reactivation. False-positive antibody responses can occur from cross-reactivity with CMV and EBV. Likewise, RF and high levels of IgG antibodies can cause false-positive and false-negative IgM test results, respectively.

Human Immunodeficiency Virus Types 1 and 2. Most infections with human immunodeficiency viruses (HIV-1 and HIV-2) are documented by serological testing. However, determination of the level of virus in serum has now become critically important for the management of infected patients. Tests initially measured the p24 antigen. However, it is now accepted that the most sensitive test is quantitative PCR. Determination of the viral load is now used to assess the response to therapy and predict the prognosis. EIA is generally used as a highly sensitive and specific screening test for antibodies directed against HIV. Most assays use viral antigens obtained from HIV-infected T-lymphocyte cell lines. The preparations are usually rich in p24, p17, gp160, gp120, and gp41 antigens. False-negative reactions can occur when the test is performed before seroconversion, when the patient is immunosuppressed, and sometimes late in the course of AIDS. Some assays that detect HIV-1 cannot detect HIV-2. The Western blot assay is the most commonly used test for confirming the presence of HIV-specific antibodies. Interpretation of the WB banding pattern varies depending on the health organization that has established the interpretive criteria.

- Food and Drug Administration: bands for p24 and p31 and for gp41, gp160, or gp120
- CDC: any two bands (p24, gp41, or gp160/120)
- American Red Cross: three or more bands with one from *gag*, *pol*, and *env*

Human T-Cell Lymphotropic Virus Types 1 and 2. Current serological procedures (e.g., IFA, LA, and EIA) cannot differentiate between human T-cell lymphotropic virus types 1 and 2 (HTLV-1 and HTLV-2). The sensitivity and specificity of EIA are >97% and >99%, respectively. Despite this, the test parameters are insufficient to permit unequivocal serodiagnosis in a low-prevalence population. Initial reactivity must be confirmed by a test such as immunoblot or RIPA. The criteria established for confirmation of HTLV-1 seropositivity include antibodies against both *env* (gp46 and/or gp61/68) and *gag* (p24) products by Western blotting or RIPA alone or in combination. A sample is considered indeterminate if antibodies against HTLV-1-specific proteins are detected in combinations other than those given above. Sera with no reactivity to any HTLV-1 proteins are considered negative or false positive. An indeterminant immunoblot is usually followed by RIPA, which has a higher sensitivity for *env* gp61/68.

Influenza Viruses. Influenza viruses can be subdivided into types (A, B, and C) by the viral nucleoprotein (NP) and matrix protein. Influenza A virus is further subdivided into subtypes by the major surface glycoproteins, hemagglutinin (HA) and neuraminidase (NA). Identification of type and subtype viruses is important for epidemiological reasons. Influenza viruses can be readily recovered in culture. Furthermore, a number of antigen-specific tests, including DFA, IFA, EIA, and RT-PCR, have been developed for influenza A virus. RT-PCR can identify type-specific and subtype-specific RNA sequences and is as sensitive as cell culture. Serological tests for influenza virus include CF, HAI, NT, and EIA. The CF test is type specific (detects antibodies to NP), develops late in infection, and is relatively insensitive. HAI measures antibodies directed against subtype-specific HA. Problems with this test include the instability of HA, the presence in patient sera of nonspecific inhibitors of hemagglutination, and the variable quality of reagents. NT is subtype specific but is performed primarily in reference laboratories. EIA can measure type- and subtype-specific antibodies of the IgG, IgM, and IgA classes.

Measles Virus. Recovery of measles virus in culture is poor and is generally less successful than for antigen tests. Measles virus antigens are detected by FA, EIA, in situ hybridization, or RT-PCR. FA and EIA are used most commonly, with hybridization and RT-PCR being restricted to research laboratories. Serological tests for measles virus include HAI, EIA, and FA. IgM and IgG antibodies generally develop within the first week of clinical disease, with a diagnostic fourfold rise in antibody titers documented 10 to 14 days later. IgM antibodies, measured by FA and EIA, develop in virtually all patients with acute infections and can provide a rapid method of documenting infection. Subacute sclerosing panencephalitis (SSPE), a neurological complication of measles virus infection, is diagnosed by demonstrating measles virus-specific antibodies in CSF. A CSF-to-serum antibody ratio of 1:5 to 1:50 is observed with this disease. The HAI test has been traditionally used to determine immunity to measles virus. However, the presence of antibodies detected by EIA indicates immunity except when active infection is suspected. Detectable immunity may not persist in vaccinated individuals.

Mumps Virus. Infection with mumps virus is documented by culture, detection of viral antigens or the viral genome, or serological testing. Virus can be isolated from saliva, urine, or CSF. DFA tests can be used to detect virus-infected cells in respiratory and CSF specimens, and the viral genome is detected by RT-PCR. Serological tests include CF, HAI, FA, and EIA. CF and HAI tests are insensitive and have been replaced with EIA. FA and EIA can be used to measure the levels of both IgM and IgG antibodies. IgM antibodies are initially detected at 5 days, peak within 1 week, and then persist for at least 6 weeks. IgG antibodies develop later and then persist for years. The presence of IgG antibodies in the absence of IgM antibodies is indicative of immunity. Cross-reactivity between mumps virus and parainfluenza virus occurs, and so antigens from both viruses must be used. IgG antibodies to mumps virus can be detected in CSF within a few days of onset of neurological disease, and peak titers are observed after 1 week.

Papillomavirus. Papillomaviruses are not grown in culture, and serological tests are not used. Infection is diagnosed by demonstration of virus-specific nucleic acids. If an effective vaccine is developed, interest in measuring the serological response to these viruses will be renewed.

Parainfluenza Virus. Parainfluenza viruses (types 1 to 4) can be cultured, but this is slow compared to antigen detection tests such as DFA, IFA, EIA, and RT-PCR. DFA and IFA are sensitive and specific and can be used to detect type-specific virus or, with pooled antibody preparations, all viruses in this group. EIAs are as specific as FA tests but less sensitive. RT-PCR is restricted primarily to research investigations. Antibodies to parainfluenza virus are detected by a variety of methods: CF, HAI, IFA, NT, and EIA.

Little experience exists with IFA tests, and NT provides results comparable to HAI; therefore, these tests are not currently used. CF is specific but insensitive. Furthermore, heterotypic response to mumps infections results in increases in antibody titers in the parainfluenza virus tests. HAI has a sensitivity comparable to CF and less than that of EIA. For these reasons, EIA is recommended for routine diagnostic use. EIA can measure IgM antibody titers, although these titers have not been found to be useful for making a rapid diagnosis or proving primary infections.

Parvovirus B19.   Parvovirus B19 has not been isolated in culture. Infection is diagnosed by electron microscopy (rarely used now), immunoassays for viral antigens or specific antibodies, and DNA-based tests. Virus can be detected by PCR tests after a week of infection, with peak viral levels occurring at 2 to 3 weeks. Immunoblotting can also be used but is less sensitive than PCR. IgM antibodies develop in the second week of infection and are detectable for 4 to 6 months. IgG antibodies develop within several days of the IgM response and persist for years. IgM antibodies can be detected in 50% of infected fetuses, and so a negative serological test does not exclude disease. Additionally, immunocompromised patients may not have detectable antibodies to parvovirus B19. Therefore, a negative serological response does not exclude infection. EIAs are commercially available for both IgM and IgG antibodies. IFA and RIA are also available for measuring antibody response.

Polyomavirus.   Two polyomaviruses cause human disease: JC virus (which causes progressive multifocal leukoencephalopathy [PML]) and BK virus (which causes urinary tract infections ranging from cystitis to fatal interstitial nephritis). The viruses can be detected in infected cells by immunofluorescence or PCR amplification of viral DNA. PCR is rapidly becoming widely available and is the method of choice. ELISAs with urine specimens are also available. HAI and ELISA are available for measuring antibodies against JC and BK viruses. However, the tests are not useful because most patients have preexisting antibodies.

Rabies Virus.   Infection with rabies virus is typically diagnosed by examining specimens (salivary cells, cutaneous

Immunodiagnostic Tests

nerves, and tissues) by DFA. Histological stains for viral inclusions (Negri bodies) are less sensitive and cannot be used to exclude the disease. Likewise, ELISAs are insensitive and nonspecific. RT-PCR is available but is no more sensitive than the FA test. Serological testing is not used for diagnostic purposes or to assess the response to vaccination (all patients respond). However, serological testing can be used to determine the immune status of individuals at continual risk of exposure to rabies. ELISAs are available for this purpose.

Respiratory Syncytial Virus. Infection with respiratory syncytial virus (RSV) can be documented by culture, DFA, IFA, EIA for viral antigen, RT-PCR, and serological testing. Culture for RSV is performed in most virology laboratories, but antigen-based tests can confirm the infection more rapidly. FA tests are also considered more sensitive than culture. The most frequently used antigen tests are EIAs. EIAs offer the advantage that intact infected cells are not needed (in contrast with FA tests). RT-PCR is restricted primarily to reference laboratories at present. Serological tests include NT, IF, EIA, and immunoblotting. Neutralizing antibodies are detected 10 days after onset of infection, peak at 3 to 4 weeks, and then decline over a 12-month period. The test is insensitive, with no antibodies detected in as many as 40% of infected individuals (particularly infants). IF tests can detect IgG, IgM, and IgA antibodies, with IgM detected within 1 week of onset and IgG detected 2 to 3 weeks later. IgA antibodies are detectable only in low concentrations. EIAs are similar to IF tests but less labor-intensive. Immunoblotting is used primarily in research laboratories.

Rhinovirus. Rhinovirus infections are documented by culture or RT-PCR (primarily a research technique). Detection of viral antigens by FA or EIA and viral antibodies by various serological tests has been complicated by the large number of viral serotypes.

Rotavirus. Rotavirus infections were first documented by immune electron microscopy. Although this method is still used in some laboratories, it has been replaced with EIA or LA in most laboratories. LA is less sensitive but is rapid and can be used at the onset of disease, when large numbers of viral particles are present in stools. Negative LA assays should be confirmed by EIA. Although PCR amplification of viral genomes and tests for antibodies against rotaviruses have been developed, these tests are restricted primarily to research laboratories.

Rubella Virus. Culture for rubella virus is slow and expensive. For this reason, serological tests have been used to document viral infections, as well as immunity to rubella. A variety of tests have been developed, including CF, passive hemagglutination (PHA), radial hemolysis (RH), LA, HAI, EIA, and IFA. The greatest experience exists with the HAI test. Detection of antibodies at a serum dilution of 1:8 (or 10 to 15 IU in the EIA) is consistent with past or current infection. IgG antibodies measured by HAI are initially detected at the time of the rash, peak at 3 weeks, and persist at detectable levels for life. Similar results are obtained with EIA, FA, and LA. PHA antibody levels peak at the same time but are lower and do not persist beyond 1 year. FA tests and EIA can be used to measure IgM and IgG antibody titers. The presence of IgM antibodies is consistent with a current infection. In the absence of IgM antibodies and because IgG antibodies persist at different levels following primary infection, a fourfold or greater increase in IgG antibody levels must be demonstrated to document active infection.

St. Louis Encephalitis Virus. A positive FA titer is $\geq 1:10$. A fourfold or greater rise in titer indicates active or recent disease.

Varicella-Zoster Virus. Infections with varicella-zoster virus (VZV) can be documented by isolation of virus in culture or detection in infected cells by DFA, electron microscopy, hybridization with DNA probes, or PCR. DFA is a practical, rapid diagnostic method if adequate numbers of infected cells are collected from the base of the vesicle. Viral culture is insensitive because the enveloped virus is labile, highly cell associated, and not shed in large numbers in older skin lesions. PCR is currently performed primarily in research laboratories but will probably become the diagnostic method of choice. Serological testing is performed either to assess immunity or to document current infection. Serological tests include CF, IFA, ACIF, EIA, and LA. CF is insensitive and is no longer used. IFAs measure the antibody response to viral membrane antigens (also called FAMA tests). These tests can identify IgM, IgG, or IgA antibodies. ACIF are preferred over IFA for technical reasons. Commercially available EIAs are now available and, although variations in test accuracy have been observed among the tests, are currently in widespread use. Antibodies first appear within a few days of the onset of the vesicular rash and peak at 2 to 3 weeks. Active disease is documented by demonstrating a fourfold rise in antibody titer. Patients with active HSV infections will produce VZV antibody rises, so that dual testing would be indicated. The LA test is a rapid, inexpensive method for demonstrating IgG antibodies in immune patients. Serum is tested at 1:4 and 1:50 dilutions (the higher dilution will detect patients with a prozone). Agglutination at either dilution indicates immunity. IgM antibodies are not detected by this test.

Western Equine Encephalitis Virus. A positive FA titer is ≥1:10. A fourfold or greater rise in antibody titer indicates active or recent infection.

Fungi

Aspergillus **Species.** EIA and RIA for *Aspergillus* antigens and CF, CIE, and ID tests for antibodies have been developed. Antigen tests are used primarily to diagnose invasive aspergillosis. Commercial EIAs detect galactomannan (GM) in serum and urine. The tests have a sensitivity between 71 and 95% (higher when monoclonal antibodies are used) and good specificity. A latex test measuring GM in serum only has also been developed but is less sensitive than EIA. The RIA is not commercially available. Antibody tests are most sensitive for immunocompetent patients with allergic bronchopulmonary aspergillosis (ABPA), pulmonary aspergilloma, and invasive aspergillosis (IA). The sensitivities of the ID and CIE tests are comparable, while ID is more specific. The CF test is more specific but less sensitive than ID. The sensitivity of ID is improved by the use of multiple antigens from *A. fumigatus*, *A. flavus*, *A. niger*, and *A. terreus*. Precipitins are present in more than 90% of patients with aspergillomas, 70% of patients with ABPA, and fewer patients with IA. A fourfold concentration of serum and retesting is recommended for patients with suspected IA and a negative ID result. The ID is highly specific, with false-positive precipitins developing only against C-reactive protein. A complement fixation antibody titer of $\geq$1:8 is considered positive.

***Blastomyces dermatitidis* (Blastomycosis).** ID, EIA, CF, and RIA have been developed for the detection of antibodies against *B. dermatitidis*. The use of the A antigen, obtained from yeast culture filtrates, has improved the specificity of these tests. The commercially available EIA is more sensitive but less specific than ID. An EIA titer of 1:32 or greater is considered diagnostic for blastomycosis. Titers 1:8 to 1:16 should be confirmed with ID or culture because cross-reactivity with *Histoplasma* antibodies can occur at this level. ID has a sensitivity of approximately 80% and a specificity approaching 100%. Antibodies are detected within 1 month of onset, and the level will decline with successful treatment. RIA has a sensitivity and specificity similar to ID but is rarely used. A CF antibody titer of $\geq$1:8 is considered positive. This test is relatively insensitive and nonspecific for blastomycosis and has generally been replaced with EIA and ID.

***Candida* Species (Candidiasis).** LA, ID, and CIE tests for antibodies and EIAs for antigens have been developed for the diagnosis of candidiasis. Antibody tests are useful for immunocompetent patients but are insensitive for patients with impaired antibody response. For this latter group of patients, antigen tests may be more useful. Antibody reactivity is detected in patients with persistent candidemia or long-standing invasive disease. Detection of a precipitin band(s) or seroconversion is consistent with systemic disease. An LA titer of 1:8 or greater or a 1:4 titer with ID precipitin bands is considered presumptive evidence of systemic disease. A 1:4 titer without a positive ID test should be repeated. ID, CIE, and LA tests have a sensitivity of about 80% for immunocompetent patients. CIE and ID are more specific than LA, which reacts in patients with infections caused by other yeasts and mycobacteria. Detection of *Candida* cell wall mannan is useful for the diagnosis of candidiasis in immunocompromised patients. The test is reported to have a specificity approaching 100% but a sensitivity only slightly greater than 50%.

***Coccidioides immitis* (Coccidioidomycosis).** CF, TP, ID, and EIA have been developed for detection of antibodies against *C. immitis*. The test antigens, called coccidioidin, are prepared from filtrates of mycelial cultures. Two primary antigens are used: a heat-stable 120-kDa glycoprotein (factor 2 antigen) located in the walls of arthroconidia and spherules, and a heat-labile 110-kDa chitinase enzyme (F antigen). The former protein is detected in the TP test, and the latter is detected in the CF test. Both antigens can be detected in the ID test and EIAs. Another antigen, spherulin, is prepared from spherules of *C. immitis* and has been used in CF tests. Factor 2 antigen is not specific for *C. immitis* and is also found in morphologically similar saprophytic fungi. The TP test is used to detect early disease (80% positive at 2 to 3 weeks, disappearing by 6 months), and the CF test detects persistent antibodies. TP remains positive in patients with disseminated disease. The combination of CF and TP tests is positive in more than 90% of infected patients. ID is comparable to CF and TP. The commercially prepared EIA measures both IgM and IgG antibodies. Both tests must be performed for maximum sensitivity. A positive EIA result must be confirmed by ID. CF antibody titers of 1:2 to 1:4 usually indicate early, residual, or meningeal disease. Antibody titers of ≥1:16 indicate disseminated disease. Negative titers do not exclude the disease.

***Cryptococcus neoformans* (Cryptococcosis).** Cryptococcal antigens can be measured by LA and EIA. EIA is more sensitive for the capsular glucuronoxylomannan polysaccharide but is technically more cumbersome. For this reason, LA remains the test of choice. Titers in serum or CSF of 1:8 or greater are considered diagnostic. Titers of 1:4 or less may be indicative of early disease or nonspecific reactions (common in patients with severe rheumatoid arthritis). Nonspecific reactions in the LA test can be eliminated by pretreating the specimen with pronase or by boiling. This is unnecessary for EIA. Other causes of false-positive reactions include contamination of specimens with syneresis fluid from condensation on agar surfaces, with disinfectants and soaps, and with *Trichosporon beigelii*. More than 99% of patients with culture-confirmed cryptococcosis have positive antigen tests. IFA, EIA, and TA have been developed for measuring cryptococcal antibodies. These tests are positive for approximately half of patients with disease and have a specificity between 77 and 89%. Because the tests have poor sensitivity and specificity, they are rarely used.

***Histoplasma capsulatum* (Histoplasmosis).**   CF, EIA, LA, and ID have been developed to measure antibodies to *H. capsulatum*, and RIA has been used to detect *Histoplasma* antigens. The CF test is sensitive (more than 90% of culture confirmed patients develop antibodies), but cross-reactions can occur in patients with blastomycosis, coccidioidomycosis, other mycoses, and leishmaniasis. Two antigens are used in the CF test: yeast phase antigen and mycelial phase antigen (also called histoplasmin). CF antibodies develop within 4 weeks after exposure in patients with pulmonary infections, with antibodies against the yeast phase being detected first and those against histoplasmin developing later. Patients with chronic histoplasmosis generally have higher titers to histoplasmin. Antibody titers between 1:8 and 1:32 are considered presumptive evidence of histoplasmosis; however, even higher titers can be observed with other diseases and should be confirmed by culture. A highly sensitive EIA has been developed, but it suffers from nonspecific reactions with other fungi. If this test is used, it must be confirmed by ID tests. The ID test can detect as many as six precipitin bands when histoplasmin is used as the test antigen. Two bands, H and M, have diagnostic value. The M band generally appears first and is an indicator of early disease. The presence of both the M and H bands is indicative of active disease, past disease, or recent skin testing. The presence of both M and H bands is consistent with active disease. The LA test is used to detect acute histoplasmosis, with reactivity occurring 2 to 3 weeks after exposure. Positive reactivity should be confirmed with the ID test. A heat-stable polysaccharide antigen can also be detected in serum, urine, and CSF specimens in patients with disseminated histoplasmosis (90% sensitivity), as well as localized pulmonary disease (<50% sensitivity). The urine test is the most sensitive for disseminated disease, but false-positive reactions have been reported with other diseases (e.g., coccidioidomycosis, paracoccidioidomycosis, penicilliosis, and blastomycosis). Positive reactions should be confirmed with culture.

Paracoccidioides brasiliensis.   CF, ID, EIA, and CIE have been developed to measure antibodies to *P. brasiliensis*. The CF test detects antibodies (titer of 1:32 or greater) in at least 80 to 95% of patients with paracoccidioidomycosis,

Immunodiagnostic Tests

while positive serological test results are reported for 98% of patients when both the CF and ID tests are used. Cross-reactivity with *H. capsulatum* can occur in the CF test. Declining CF titers are consistent with a response to therapy, and the presence of persistently high titers indicates a bad prognosis. One to three unique precipitin bands are observed in the ID test. Antigen 1 has been characterized as a 43-kDa glycoprotein. This antigen has also been used in EIA. Both the CF and ID tests are available through the CDC.

***Penicillium marneffei* (Penicilliosis).** The presence of a precipitin band(s) indicates a positive ID assay. Data regarding the sensitivity and specificity of this test are not currently available. The test should be used to confirm the clinical diagnosis of penicilliosis. These infections are usually disseminated, with multiple-organ involvement including lymphadenitis, subcutaneous abscesses, bone lesions, arthritis, splenomegaly, and lesions in the lung, liver, or bowel. The diagnostic test of choice is recovery of *P. marneffei* in clinical specimens.

***Pneumocystis carinii* (Pneumocystosis).** *P. carinii* grows poorly in cell culture, and reliable antigen or antibody tests have not been developed. Demonstration of the organism in clinical specimens by microscopy is diagnostic. Toluidine blue O, calcofluor white, and methenamine silver stain the cyst wall; Gram and Papanicolaou stains stain the trophozoite forms; and Giemsa and fluorescein-labeled antibodies (DFA) stain both cysts and trophozoites.

***Sporothrix schenckii* (Sporotrichosis).** EIA, LA, and TA can be used reliably to detect antibodies to *S. schenckii*, while the CF and ID tests are less reliable and are not recommended. Antibodies to at least two cell wall antigens (40- and 70-kDa antigens) are detected. EIA titers of at least 1:16 in serum and 1:8 in CSF are considered diagnostic. Elevated titers can be observed, which decline with successful therapy. LA titers of 1:4 or greater are consistent with disease, although nonspecific reactions can occur at titers of 1:8. Antibody titers in the LA test do not change predictably with therapy, so they cannot be used for prognostic purposes.

Zygomycetes (Zygomycosis, Mucomycosis). EIA and ID have been developed to detect antibodies in patients with active zygomycosis. The tests have a sensitivity of approximately 70% and a specificity of greater than 90%. They are rarely used because the etiologic agents of zygomycosis grow rapidly.

Parasites

***Babesia microti* (Babesiosis).**   Babesiosis is diagnosed by observation of parasitized erythrocytes. However, in patients with low-grade parasitemia or inconclusive peripheral smears, serological testing can be helpful. Antibody titers in the IFA test rise rapidly during the first weeks of disease to 1:1,024 or higher and then gradually decline over the next 6 months. Low but detectable titers may persist for 1 year or more. Elevated antibody titers may be present in healthy individuals in areas of endemic infection. Therefore, a positive serological test result should be confirmed by detection of the parasite in blood smears. Cross-reactivity among *Babesia* species is variable, so regional differences in serological reactivity may be observed.

Cryptosporidium parvum.   Cryptosporidiosis is diagnosed by observation of the parasite in clinical specimens (e.g., traditional microscopic techniques, DFA, and IFA) or detection of specific antigens by EIA. Both the microscopic methods and EIA have high sensitivity and specificity.

***Echinococcus* Species (Echinococcosis).**   Serological tests to confirm the clinical diagnosis of echinococcosis should be performed before invasive procedures are used. IHA, IFA, and EIA have been used to confirm cystic hydatid disease (CHD) caused by *E. granulosus*. The test sensitivity ranges from 60 to 90% and is improved when a combination of tests is used. Antibody reactivity in patients is influenced by the location and integrity of the cyst. Detectable antibodies are more common in patients with cysts in the bones and liver than in those with cysts in the lungs, brain, and spleen. Seroreactivity is always lower in patients with intact cysts. False-positive reactions may occur in persons with other helminthic infections, cancer, collagen vascular disease, and cirrhosis. EIAs are used to diagnose alveolar hydatid disease due to *E. multilocularis*. The use of purified antigens (i.e., Em2 and recombinant antigen II/3-10) improves the overall sensitivity and specificity of this test.

Immunodiagnostic Tests

***Entamoeba histolytica* (Amebiasis).** Detection of *Entamoeba histolytica* antigens in fecal specimens by EIA is generally less sensitive than is microscopic examination of the specimen. Serological testing has proven useful for patients with extraintestinal disease because amebas are not reliably seen in fecal specimens. IHA is the reference test. The CDC recommends the use of ≥1:256 as a criterion for a positive IHA serological result. This level will identify 95% of patients with extraintestinal infections, 70% of patients with active disease localized to the intestines, and 10% of asymptomatic intestinal carriers. Positive titers may persist for years after successful therapy. EIA is a sensitive assay, which identifies significantly more patients with hepatic disease than does IHA. No cross-reactions with other amebas are observed. Detection of IgM antibodies is insensitive, even for patients with active invasive disease (positive in only 65% of the patients).

Fasciola hepatica. EIAs with the excretory-secretory (ES) antigens are the tests of choice. Specific antibodies appear within 2 to 4 weeks after infection (5 to 7 weeks before eggs appear in the stool). Sensitivity approaches 95%; however, cross-reactivity may occur with serum specimens from patients with schistosomiasis. These reactions can be resolved by detecting parasite-specific 12-, 17-, and 63-kDa antigens in immunoblot assays. Antibody titers decrease rapidly following treatment and hence can be used to predict the success of therapy.

Filariae (Filariasis). Positive serum antibody tests are of little diagnostic value except in patients not native to areas of filarial endemicity. Most residents of regions where filariae are endemic have high antibody levels. Additionally, cross-reactions with other nematode parasites can occur. Serological testing may be useful for confirming a clinical diagnosis of filariasis in a traveler to an area of endemic infection.

***Giardia lamblia* (Giardiasis).** Monitoring the antibody response in *Giardia* infections is not commonly done, because the antigen can be detected by a variety of immunoassays and microscopy. A number of commercially prepared DFA tests and EIAs are available. The DFA tests detect *Giardia* cysts and reportedly have a sensitivity and specificity of 100%. The EIAs detect either cysts only or cysts and trophozoites. Purified antigens are used in most of these tests and have sensitivities and specificities greater than 95%.

***Leishmania* Species (Leishmaniasis).** The presence of genus-specific antibodies to *Leishmania* is determined by the IFA test. The sensitivity of this test is >90% for patients with visceral leishmaniasis but very low for those with cutaneous disease. Cross-reactions occur in patients with Chagas' disease.

***Paragonimus westermani* (Paragonimiasis).** Serological tests for paragonimiasis include CF, immunofluorescence, EIAs, and immunoblot assays. The tests are highly sensitive and specific. An 8-kDa antigen-antibody band was present in 96% of patients with confirmed infection, and the specificity was >99%. Antibody titers decrease rapidly after successful therapy and so can be used to monitor response.

***Plasmodium* Species (Malaria).** Serodiagnosis of malaria is recommended for screening blood donors suspected of a previous infection and for testing a patient from an area of endemic disease who has a febrile illness and negative blood smears. The test is sensitive and specific but cannot discriminate between active and past infection. The immunofluorescence test uses antigens from all four *Plasmodium* species associated with human disease.

***Schistosoma* Species (Schistosomiasis).** Test sensitivity and specificity are highly dependent upon the antigen preparation used and the testing method. ELISAs with *S. mansoni* adult microsomal antigen are sensitive for infections with this species but less so for *S. japonicum* and *S. haematobium*. The use of immunoblots ensures the detection of the other two species if the clinical history suggests these infections. Species specificity is gained in immunoblots when adult worm antigens are used.

***Strongyloides stercoralis* (Strongyloidiasis).** EIAs, with a sensitivity reported to be between 84 and 92%, are currently recommended for the diagnosis of strongyloidiasis. Immunocompromised persons typically mount a detectable immune response. Nonreactivity is observed in 8 to 16% of carriers. Cross-reactions can occur in patients with filariasis and some other nematode infections. The highest antibody sensitivity and specificity are obtained when antigens derived from *S. stercoralis* filariform larvae are used. The tests cannot differentiate between active and past infection.

***Taenia solium* (Cysticercosis).**   The immunoblot assay has a sensitivity approaching 100% and is more sensitive than other available assays. Seropositivity is reported in 50 to 70% of patients with a single cyst, 80% of patients with multiple calcified lesions, and >90% of patients with multiple noncalcified lesions. EIAs are less sensitive than the immunoblot assay and cross-react with antibodies specific for other helminth infections. Currently available tests do not distinguish between active and inactive infections, so serological testing cannot be used to evaluate the outcome or prognosis following treatment.

***Toxocara canis* (Visceral and Ocular Larva Migrans).**   Antibody tests are the only means to confirm the presumptive diagnosis of toxocaral visceral larva migrans (VLM) or ocular larva migrans (OLM). Larval antigens are used in EIAs. The test sensitivity and specificity cannot be precisely assessed because alternative methods to demonstrate infection have not been developed. However, the test sensitivity is estimated to vary from 70 to 80% and the specificity is estimated to be >90%, with a higher sensitivity for VLM.

***Toxoplasma gondii* (Toxoplasmosis).**   A number of antibody tests for toxoplasmosis are commercially available. IFA and EIA for IgG and IgM antibodies are used most commonly. Screening should be performed with an IgG test. A negative reaction indicates no infection, while a positive reaction can represent either current or past infection. If IgM antibodies are not present, the patient was infected more than 2 years previously. A positive IgG reaction and a high titer of IgM antibodies indicate a recent or current infection. The presence of a low IgM titer could indicate nonspecific reactivity. This can be resolved by repeat testing after a few weeks. The immunofluorescence test is defined as negative when the IgG antibody titer is ≤1:16 (except for ocular infections, where low titers are commonplace), equivocal at a titer of 1:16 to 1:256, and positive at a titer of >1:256. Positive response is also defined as a fourfold or greater increase in antibody titer. IgM antibody titers of ≥1:64 are indicative of active infection in adults, while any IgM antibody titer is considered significant in newborns. The sensitivity of EIA is considered equivalent to that of the immunofluorescence test. Serological determination of active central nervous system toxoplasmosis in immunocompromised patients is not possible at this time. Specific IgG antibody levels in these patients are often low, and IgM antibodies are generally nondetectable.

***Trichinella spiralis* (Trichinosis).** Detectable antibodies do not develop until 3 to 5 weeks after infection (well after the acute stage of illness), peak in the second or third month, and then decline slowly for several years. Antibodies are detected earlier with the EIA than with other test methods, but the EIA is less specific. Positive EIA results can be confirmed by flocculation tests.

***Trichomonas vaginalis* (Trichomoniasis)**. Trichomoniasis is diagnosed by detection of trophozoites by microscopic examination, DFA, or culture. Antigen-specific agglutination tests, with high sensitivity and specificity, are also available.

***Trypanosoma cruzi* (Chagas' Disease).** Diagnosis of Chagas' disease during the acute stage is based on detection of trypomastigotes in peripheral blood. The parasites are rare or absent during the chronic phase of illness, so laboratory confirmation of disease typically depends upon serological testing. IFA and EIA are available. Both tests are very sensitive, but cross-reactivity occurs in patients with leishmaniasis, a disease that occurs in the same geographical area. CF is less sensitive. An elevated antibody titer cannot be used to differentiate between active and past disease.

Immunodiagnostic Tests

Table 7.1   Criteria for diagnosis of syphilis[a]

Early syphilis

Primary

Definitive: direct microscopic identification of *T. pallidum* in lesion material, lymph node aspirate, or biopsy section

Presumptive (requires 1 and either 2 or 3)
1. Typical lesion
2. Reactive nontreponemal test and no history of syphilis
3. For persons with history of syphilis, fourfold increase in most recent quantitative nontreponemal test titer compared with results of past tests

Suggestive (requires 1 and 2)
1. Lesion resembling chancre
2. Sexual contact within preceding 90 days with person who has primary, secondary, or early latent syphilis

Secondary

Definitive: direct microscopic identification of *T. pallidum* in lesion material, lymph node aspirate, or biopsy section

Presumptive (requires 1 and either 2 or 3)
1. Skin or mucous membrane lesions typical of secondary syphilis
   a. Macular, papular, follicular, papulosquamous, or pustular
   b. Condylomata lata (anogenital region or mouth)
   c. Mucous patches (oropharynx or cervix)
2. Reactive nontreponemal test titer of ≥1:8 and no previous history of syphilis
3. For person with history of syphilis, fourfold increase in most recent nontreponemal test tier compared with previous test results

Suggestive (requires 1 and 2 and is made only when serological test results are not available)
1. Presence of clinical manifestations as described above
2. Sexual exposure within past 6 mo to person with early syphilis

Early latent

Definitive: Definitive diagnosis does not exist because lesions are not present in latent stage.

Presumptive (requires 1, 2, and 3 or 4)
1. Absence of signs and symptoms
2. Reactive nontreponemal and treponemal test results
3. Nonreactive nontreponemal test within preceding yr
4. Fourfold increase in nontreponemal test titer compared with previous test results for persons with history of syphilis or of symptoms compatible with early syphilis

Suggestive (requires 1 and 2)
1. Reactive nontreponemal test result
2. History of sexual exposure within preceding yr

(continued)

Table 7.1 Criteria for diagnosis of syphilis[a] *(continued)*

Late syphilis
Benign and cardiovascular
Definitive: observation of treponemes in tissue sections by direct microscopic examination with DFAT-TP
Presumptive
1. Reactive treponemal test
2. No known history of treatment for syphilis
3. Characteristic symptoms of benign or cardiovascular syphilis
Neurosyphilis
Definitive (requires 1 and either 2 or 3)
1. Reactive serum treponemal test
2. Reactive VDRL CSF test on spinal fluid sample
3. Identification of *T. pallidum* in CSF or tissue by microscopic examination or animal inoculation
Presumptive (requires 1 and either 2 or 3)
1. Reactive serum treponemal test
2. Clinical signs of neurosyphilis
3. Elevated CSF protein (>40 mg/dl) or leukocyte count (>5 mononuclear cells/ml) in absence of other known causes

Neonatal congenital syphilis
Definitive: demonstration of *T. pallidum* by direct microscopic examination of umbilical cord, placenta, nasal discharge, or skin lesion material
Presumptive (requires 1, 2, and 3)
1. Determination that infant was born to mother who had untreated or inadequately treated syphilis at delivery regardless of findings in infant
2. Infant with reactive treponemal test result
3. One of following additional criteria:
   a. Clinical sign or symptoms of congenital syphilis on physical examination
   b. Abnormal CSF finding without other cause
   c. Reactive VDRL CSF test result
   d. Reactive IgM antibody test specific for syphilis

---

[a]Abbreviations: CSF, cerebrospinal fluid; DFAT-TP, direct fluorescent-antibody test for *T. pallidum* with staining of tissue sections; VDRL, Venereal Disease Research Laboratory.
Source: S. J. Norris and S. A. Larsen, p. 636–651, *in* P. R. Murray, E. J. Baron, M. A. Pfaller, F. C. Tenover, and R. H. Yolken (ed.), *Manual of Clinical Microbiology*, 6th ed., American Society for Microbiology, Washington, D.C., 1995.

Table 7.2 Correlation of clinical status and characteristic serological responses to EBV infection[a]

Clinical status	Heterophile antibody (qualitative test)	EBV-specific antibodies Characteristic antibody profile[b]				
		IgM-VCA	IgG-VCA	EA-D	EA-R	EBNA
Negative reaction	Negative	<1:8[c]	<1:10	<1:10	<1:10	<1:2.5
Susceptible	−	−	−	−	−	−
Acute primary infection (infectious mononucleosis)	+	1:32 to 1:256	1:160 to 1:640	1:40 to 1:160	−[d]	− to 1:2.5
Recent primary infection (infectious mononucleosis)	±	− to 1:32	1:320 to 1:1,280	1:40 to 1:160	−[d]	1:5 to 1:10
Remote (previous) infection	−	−	1:40 to 1:160	−[e]	− to 1:40	1:10 to 1:40
Reactivation in an immunosuppressed or immunocompromised individual	−	−	1:320 to 1:1,280	−[e]	1:80 to 1:320	− to 1:160
Burkitt's lymphoma	−	−	1:320 to 1:1,280	−[e]	1:80 to 1:320	1:10 to 1:80
Nasopharyngeal carcinoma	−	−	1:320 to 1:1,280	1:40 to 1:160	−[f]	1:20 to 1:160

[a] Adapted from N. R. Rose, E. C. de Macario, J. D. Folds, H. C. Lane, and R. M. Nakamura, ed., *Manual of Clinical Laboratory Immunology*, 5th ed., ASM Press, Washington, D.C., 1997 (p. 637).
[b] Individual responses outside the characteristic range may occur. −, negative; +, positive; ±, positive or negative.
[c] Some laboratories report <1:10 as the lowest dilution tested.
[d] In young children and adults with asymptomatic seroconversion, the anti-EA response may be mainly to the EA-D component.
[e] A minority of individuals will have the anti-EA response mainly to the EA-D component.
[f] A minority of individuals will have the anti-EA response mainly to the EA-R component.

Immunodiagnostic Tests

Immunodiagnostic Tests

Table 7.3 Interpretation of HBV serological markers in patients with hepatitis[a]

Assay result[a]			Interpretation
HBsAg	Anti-HBs	Anti-HBc	
Positive	Negative	Negative	Early acute HBV infection. Confirmation is required to exclude nonrepeatable or nonspecific reactivity.
Positive	(±)[b]	Positive	HBV infection, either acute or chronic. Differentiate with IgM anti-HBc. Determine level of infectivity with HBeAg or HBV DNA.
Negative	Positive	Positive	Indicates previous HBV infection and immunity to hepatitis B.
Negative	Negative	Positive	Possibilities include HBV infection in remote past, "low-level" HBV carrier, "window" between disappearance of HBsAg and appearance of anti-HBs, or false-positive reaction. Investigate with IgM anti-HBc and/or challenge with HBsAg vaccine. When present, anti-HBe helps validate anti-HBc reactivity.
Negative	Negative	Negative	Another infectious agent, toxic injury to liver, disorder of immunity, hereditary disease of liver, or disease of biliary tract
Negative	Positive	Negative	Vaccine-type response

[a] Abbreviations: Anti-HBs, antibodies to hepatitis B surface antigen; HBc, antibodies to hepatitis B core antigen; HBe, antibodies to hepatitis e antigen; HBeAg, hepatitis e antigen; HBsAg, hepatitis B surface antigen.

[b] ±, Anti-HBs is usually absent in this situation but may occasionally be present.

Source: F. B. Hollinger and J. L. Dienstag, p. 1033–1049, *in* P. R. Murray, E. J. Baron, M. A. Pfaller, F. C. Tenover, and R. H. Yoken. ed., *Manual of Clinical Microbiology*, 6th ed., ASM Press, Washington, D.C., 1995.

Notifiable Infectious Diseases

National notification is required for 49 infectious diseases, which are reported on a weekly basis in the Centers for Disease Control and Prevention *Morbidity and Mortality Weekly Report* (MMWR). Although these reports are useful for tracking the prevalence and geographic distribution of specific diseases, their accuracy is dependent on the diagnostic tests that are used and the diligence with which physicians, microbiologists, hospital administrators, and public health officials report the diseases. Data reported for some diseases, such as anthrax, plague, and rabies, are assumed to be accurate because the diseases are uncommon and generate a high level of public interest. Other diseases are reported less reliably because specific diagnostic tests may not be performed (e.g., *Chlamydia trachomatis* infections in males) or may be inaccurate (e.g., tests for Lyme disease or legionellosis). Additionally, trend analysis must be analyzed carefully because the definition of disease, diagnostic tests, or reporting criteria may be changed. For example, the case definition used for AIDS was modified in 1993, and this affected the incidence data.

Nationally Notifiable Infectious Diseases—1997[a]

AIDS (human immunodeficiency virus; 56,492)

AIDS (pediatric infections; 231)

Anthrax (*Bacillus anthracis*; 0)

Botulism (*Clostridium botulinum*; 105[b])

Brucellosis (*Brucella* spp.; 76)

Chlamydia (*C. trachomatis* genital infection; 467,792)

Cholera (*Vibrio cholerae*; 10)

Coccidioidomycosis (*Coccidioides immitis*; data not available)

Cryptosporidiosis (*Cryptosporidium parvum*; 1963)

Diphtheria (*Corynebacterium diphtheriae*; 5)

Encephalitis, California (120)

Encephalitis, eastern equine (10)

Encephalitis, St. Louis (12)

Encephalitis, western equine (0)

(continued)

Escherichia coli O157:H7 (2,316)

Hemolytic-uremic syndrome (postdiarrheal; 61)

Chancroid (*Haemophilus ducreyi*; 386[b])

Gonorrhea (*Neisseria gonorrhoeae*; 289,870)

Haemophilus influenzae infections (invasive infections; 1,056)

Hantavirus pulmonary syndrome (18)

Hepatitis A (27,799)

Hepatitis B (8,749)

Hepatitis C/non-A, non-B (3,164)

Legionellosis (*Legionella* spp.; 1,054)

Leprosy (*Mycobacterium leprae* [Hansen's disease]; 109)

Lyme disease (*Borrelia burgdorferi*; 10,979)

Malaria (*Plasmodium* spp.; 1,772)

Measles (rubeola; 135)

Mumps (612)

Neisseria meningitidis infections (disseminated; 3,117)

Pertussis (*Bordetella pertussis*; 5,519)

Plague (*Yersinia pestis*; 4)

Poliomyelitis (paralytic; 1)

Psittacosis (*Chlamydia psittaci*; 37)

Rabies (animal; 7,853)

Rabies (human; 2)

Rocky Mountain spotted fever (*Rickettsia rickettsii*; 400)

Rubella (German measles; 161)

Rubella (congenital; 4)

Salmonellosis (*Salmonella* spp.; 45,471[b])

Shigellosis (*Shigella* spp.; 25,978[b])

Streptococcal disease (invasive group A *Streptococcus* disease; 1,431)

Streptococcus pneumoniae infections (penicillin-resistant strains; data not available)

Syphilis (congenital; 548)

Syphilis (all stages; 52,976[b])

Tetanus (*Clostridium tetani*; 43)

Toxic shock syndrome (staphylococcal; 134)

Toxic shock syndrome (streptococcal; 33)

Trichinosis (*Trichinella spirilis*; 9)

Tuberculosis (*Mycobacterium tuberculosis*; 17,158)

Typhoid fever (*Salmonella typhi*; 346)

Yellow fever (0)

---

[a]Data from *Morbid. Mortal. Weekly Rep.* **46**:1265–1269, 1998; numbers in parentheses represent the number of cases reported in 1997.
[b]Data from 1996.

Geographic Distribution of Selected Notifiable Diseases—Totals for 1992–1996

AIDS (365,874)
New York (65,587), California (60,108), Florida (40,038), Texas (25,649), New Jersey (20,489), Illinois (12,394), Pennsylvania (11,793), Maryland (11,282), Georgia (11,060)

Botulism (533)
California (169), Alaska (43), Texas (39), Pennsylvania (33), Washington (26), New Jersey (24)

Brucellosis (554)
California (155), Texas (132), North Carolina (54), Illinois (31), Arizona (25), Florida (23)

Chancroid (4,990)
New York (2,322), Louisiana (1,047), Texas (498), Illinois (305), Florida (189), Arkansas (172 [170 in 1993]), North Carolina (93)

Cholera (187)
California (97), Nevada (15 [all in 1992]), Texas (13), New York (10), Florida (6)

Gonorrhea (2,077,881)
Texas (149,962), New York (141,478), California (137,989), Georgia (129,736), Illinois (123,875), North Carolina (121,680), Florida (116,254), Ohio (112,919)

Haemophilus influenzae Infection (Invasive Disease; 6,355)
California (926), Ohio (544), New York (460), Maryland (370), Georgia (327), Missouri (303 [216 in 1992–1993]), Illinois (251), Pennsylvania (225), Minnesota (205)

Hepatitis A (136,760)
California (30,619), Texas (13,964), Arizona (8,007), Missouri (6,314), New York (5,947), Oregon (5,921), Oklahoma (4,864), Washington (4,846), Ohio (4,535)

Hepatitis B (63,446)
California (10,189), Texas (6,785), New York (4,435), Tennessee (4,410), Florida (3,860), Missouri (2,421), Michigan (2,223)

Hepatitis C/non-A, non-B (23,558)

Tennessee (4,535), California (3,161), Michigan (1,689), Texas (1,562), New York (1,314), Louisiana (1,034)

Leprosy (751)

California (268), Texas (179), Hawaii (92), New York (54), Washington (34), Massachusetts (28), Florida (15)

Legionellosis (6,673)

Ohio (773), Pennsylvania (715), New York (451), California (376), Michigan (359), Florida (278), Indiana (266), Maryland (245)

Lyme Disease (59,350)

New York (21,202), Connecticut (9,792), Pennsylvania (8,072), New Jersey (6,900), Wisconsin (2,100), Maryland (1,605)

Malaria (6,946)

California (1,321), New York (1,294), Texas (416), Maryland (344), Florida (335), New Jersey (303), Illinois (282)

Neisseria meningitidis Infection (Invasive Disease; 14,337)

California (1,839), Texas (976), Florida (795), New York (772), Oregon (593), Ohio (589), Illinois (580), Pennsylvania (578)

Pertussis (28,219)

Massachusetts (3,122), California (3,045), New York (2,078), Washington (1,793), Wisconsin (1,342), Ohio (1,268), Pennsylvania (1,223), Colorado (1,011)

Plague (54)

New Mexico (23), Arizona (12), California (6), Colorado (5), Utah (3), Idaho, Nevada, Oregon, Texas, and Wyoming (1 each)

Psittacosis (296)

California (43), Washington (31), Pennsylvania (28), New York (26), Oregon (16), Ohio (12), Wisconsin (11)

Rabies (Animal; 40,906)

New York (8,228), Connecticut (3,002), Maryland (2,754), Texas (2,514), Virginia (2,248), Massachusetts (2,027), New Jersey (1,928), Pennsylvania (1,899), California (1,862), Georgia (1,802)

Notifiable Diseases

(continued)

Rabies (Human; 18)

California (5), Florida (2), Texas (2), Alabama, Connecticut, Kentucky, Montana, New Hampshire, New York, Tennessee, Washington, and West Virginia (1 each)

Rocky Mountain Spotted Fever (2,844)

North Carolina (726), Oklahoma (273), Georgia (215), Tennessee (191), Virginia (150), Maryland (125), Missouri (115), Arkansas (112)

Salmonellosis (217,307)

California (31,288), New York (19,622), Florida (14,428), Texas (11,003), Pennsylvania (10,369), Illinois (9,823), Massachusetts (9,238), Georgia (7,545)

Shigellosis (143,956)

California (24,215), Texas (16,333), Florida (10,559), New York (7,636), Illinois (6,501), North Carolina (6,302), Georgia (5,406), Arizona (4,923), Pennsylvania (4,006)

Syphilis (Congenital; 11,975)

New York (2,484), Illinois (1,246), California (1,205), Texas (1,114), Florida (835), Pennsylvania (678), New Jersey (642)

Syphilis (All Stages; 417,465)

New York (53,343), Texas (43,553), California (36,496), Florida (27,148), Louisiana (24,944), Illinois (20,774), Georgia (19,844), North Carolina (19,422), Mississippi (19,177)

Tetanus (221)

Texas (30), California (29), Florida (17), Michigan (13), New York (12), Minnesota (11), Illinois (8)

Tuberculosis (120,544)

California (24,443), New York (17,787), Texas (11,920), Florida (8,097), Illinois (5,713), New Jersey (4,419), Georgia (3,979), Pennsylvania (3,382), North Carolina (2,837), Tennessee (2,572)

Typhoid Fever (2,060)

California (509), New York (438), Florida (135), New Jersey (135), Illinois (131), Massachusetts (112), Texas (86)

Notifiable Diseases

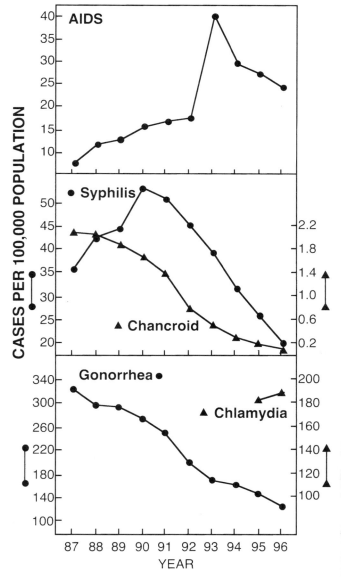

Figure 8.1 AIDS, syphilis, chancroid, gonorrhea, and *Chlamydia*.

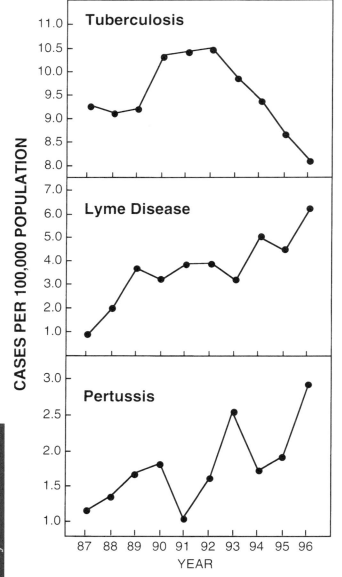

Figure 8.2 Tuberculosis, Lyme disease, and pertussis.

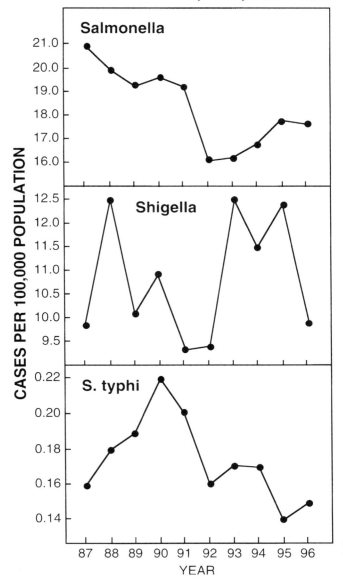

Figure 8.3 *Salmonella, Shigella,* and *S. typhi.*

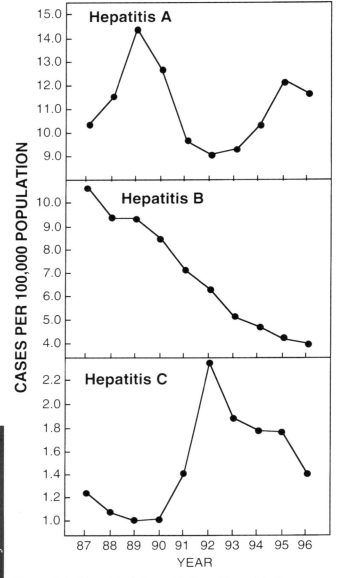

Figure 8.4 Hepatitis A, hepatitis B, and hepatitis C.

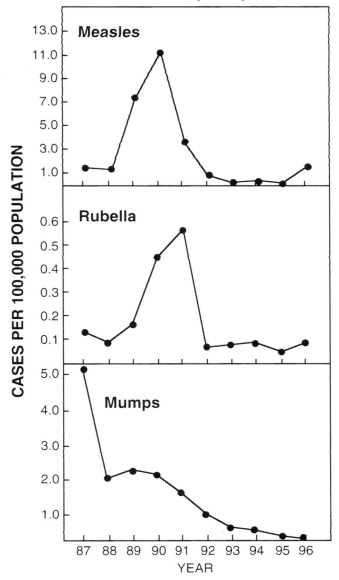

Figure 8.5 Measles, rubella, and mumps.

Bibliography

For additional information regarding the subjects discussed in this pocket guide, please refer to the following general reference texts.

Ash, L. R., and T. C. Orihel. 1997. *Atlas of Human Parasitology*, 4th ed. American Society of Clinical Pathologists, Chicago, Ill.

Atlas, R., and L. Parks. 1993. *Handbook of Microbiological Media*. CRC Press, Inc., Boca Raton, Fla.

Balows, A., H. Trüper, M. Dworkin, W. Harder, and K. H. Schleifer. 1992. *The Prokaryotes*, 2nd ed. Springer-Verlag, New York, N.Y.

Collier, L., A. Balows, and M. Sussman. 1998. *Topley & Wilson's Microbiology and Microbial Infections*, 9th ed. Edward Arnold, London, United Kingdom.

Forbes, B. A., D. F. Sahm, and A. S. Weissfeld. 1998. *Bailey & Scott's Diagnostic Microbiology*, 10th ed. Mosby-Year Book, Inc., St. Louis, Mo.

Garcia, L. S., and D. A. Bruckner. 1997. *Diagnostic Medical Parasitology*, 3rd ed. American Society for Microbiology, Washington, D.C.

Holt, J., N. Krieg, P. Sneath, J. Staley, and S. Williams. 1994. *Bergey's Manual of Determinative Bacteriology*, 9th ed. The Williams & Wilkins Co., Baltimore, Md.

Isenberg, H. 1992. *Clinical Microbiology Procedures Handbook*. American Society for Microbiology, Washington, D.C.

Kucers, A., and N. M. Bennett. 1989. *The Use of Antibiotics*, 4th ed. J. B. Lippincott Co., Philadelphia, Pa.

Kwon-Chung, K., and J. Bennett. 1992. *Medical Mycology*. Lea & Febiger, Philadelphia, Pa.

Larone, D. 1995. *Medically Important Fungi–a Guide to Identification*, 3rd ed. American Society for Microbiology, Washington, D.C.

Mandell, G., J. Bennett, and R. Dolin. 1995. *Principles and Practice of Infectious Diseases*, 4th ed. Churchill Livingstone, Inc., New York, N.Y.

Miller, J. M. 1996. *A Guide to Specimen Management in Clinical Microbiology.* American Society for Microbiology, Washington, D.C.

Murray, P. R., E. J. Baron, M. A. Pfaller, F. C. Tenover, and R. H. Yolken. 1995. *Manual of Clinical Microbiology*, 6th ed. American Society for Microbiology, Washington, D.C.

Murray, P. R., K. S. Rosenthal, G. S. Kobayashi, and M. A. Pfaller. 1998. *Medical Microbiology*, 3rd ed. Mosby-Year Book, Inc., St. Louis, Mo.

Rose, N. R., E. Conway de Macario, J. D. Folds, H. C. Lane, and R. M. Nakamura. 1997. *Manual of Clinical Laboratory Immunology*, 5th ed. American Society for Microbiology, Washington, D.C.

Schreckenberger, P. C. 1996. *Practical Approach to the Identification of Glucose-Nonfermenting Gram-Negative Bacilli: a Guide to Identification.* Colorado Association for Continuing Medical Laboratory Education, Inc., Denver.

St. Germain, G., and R. Summerbell. 1996. *Identifying Filamentous Fungi: a Clinical Laboratory Handbook.* Star Publishing Co., Belmont, Calif.

Summanen, P., E. Baron, D. Citron, C. Strong, H. Wexler, and S. Finegold. 1993. *Wadsworth Anaerobic Bacteriology Manual*, 5th ed. Star Publishing Co., Belmont, Calif.

Weyant, R. S., C. W. Moss, R. E. Weaver, D. G. Hollis, J. G. Jordan, E. C. Cook, and M. I. Daneshvar. 1995. *Identification of Unusual Pathogenic Gram-Negative Aerobic and Facultatively Anaerobic Bacteria*, 2nd ed. The Williams & Wilkins Co., Baltimore, Md.

Index

Staphylococcus aureus, 34, 37–45, 47–50, 52–53, 129, 178

Stavudine, 255, 266, 287

Stenotrophomonas, 4, 203, 206, 281

Stomatococcus, 8, 34, 43, 177, 179–180, 274

Stool specimen
amebae and flagellate, 224
ciliates, coccidia, and *Blastocystis*, 227
flagellates, 233

Streptobacillus, 90, 281

Streptococcal disease, 333

Streptococcus, 5, 34–35, 37–45, 48, 50–53, 83–84, 129, 179, 181–182, 271, 274–275, 305, 333
group A, see *Streptococcus pyogenes*
group B, see *Streptococcus agalactiae*
viridans group, 43, 47, 52–53, 84, 182, 275

Streptococcus agalactiae, 34, 40, 45, 51–52, 83, 181, 305

Streptococcus pneumoniae, 35, 37–39, 41, 43–45, 50, 52–53, 83, 271, 275, 305, 333

Streptococcus pyogenes, 35, 37–39, 43, 53, 83, 129, 181, 305

Streptomycin, 255, 266, 283

Strongyloides, 40, 50, 76, 105, 174, 238, 291, 324

Strongyloidiasis, 324

Succinivibrio, 35

Sucking lice, 242

Sulfadiazine, 266

Sulfadoxine, 266

Sulfadoxine-pyrimethamine, 255

Sulfamethizole, 266

Sulfamethoxazole, 266

Sulfisoxazole, 255, 267

Sulfonamides, 289

Suramin, 290

Suttonella, 5, 200

Synovial fluid specimen
collection and transport, 116–117
processing, 158, 161

Syphilis, 333, 336–337
criteria for diagnosis, 327–328

T

Taenia, 18, 80, 106, 172, 236, 239, 325

Tapeworms, 290

Teicoplanin, 267

Terbinafine, 256, 289

Termites, 241–242

Tetanus, 333, 336

Tetracycline, 256, 267, 282, 290

Tetrathionate broth, 143

Thayer-Martin (modified) agar, 143

Thiabendazole, 256, 290–291

Thioglycolate broth, 143

Thiosulfate citrate bile salts sucrose agar, 143–144

Thoracentesis fluid, specimen processing, 158, 161

Throat specimen, collection and transport, 125

Thymol blue, 150

Ticarcillin, 256, 267

Ticarcillin-clavulanate, 256, 267, 277

Ticks, 19, 55, 241

Tinsdale agar, 144

Tissierella, 35

Tissue specimen
collection and transport, 125–126
processing, 160, 163

Tobramycin, 256, 267

Toluidine blue-O stain, 157

Torovirus, 49

Toxic shock syndrome, 333

Toxocara, 17, 53–55, 76, 238, 291, 325

Toxoplasma, 16, 40, 44–45, 47–48, 54–55, 72, 105, 171–172, 174, 226, 290, 325–326

Toxoplasmosis, 325–326

Tracheal specimen
collection and transport, 122
processing, 159, 163

Trachipleistophora, 17, 73

Transfusion-associated sepsis, 45, 165

Transtracheal aspirate, specimen processing, 159, 163

Trematodes, 76–80, 106–107, 173, 240, 291

Trench fever, 56

Treponema, 9, 35, 45–46, 48, 51, 54, 92, 283, 327–328

NOTES

NOTES

NOTES

NOTES

NOTES

NOTES

NOTES

NOTES

NOTES